Low Cholesterol Recipes

Superfoods and Gluten Free that <u>May</u> Lower Cholesterol

Tracy Prior

Table of Contents

Low Cholesterol Recipes
Introduction

The low cholesterol diet has been around for a long time, and really there is no "one" diet that can stake the claim as the only low cholesterol diet. Many physicians, however, including the American Heart Association, recommend eating a diet that is naturally low in bad cholesterol for the sake of losing weight and to help manage cholesterol levels and to treat conditions caused by high cholesterol levels in the body.

Here is a quick overview of different cholesterol levels. First, when testing for cholesterol levels there are three readings that constitute the levels - the "total cholesterol" and the LDL (the unfavorable cholesterol and the HDL (the good cholesterol. A blood test will give number readings for these. For the HDL cholesterol one that is too low is lower than 40 and one that is too high is higher than 60. The LDL cholesterol has five different levels. Very high is above a 190, high is 160-189, borderline high is 130-159, above optimal is 100-129 with optimal being 100 or lower. Total cholesterol has three levels with high being greater than a 240, borderline high being 200-239 and normal is less than 200.

The main purpose of going on a "low cholesterol" diet is to lower the levels of blood cholesterol test, especially the LDL. LDL cholesterol is the type that causes plaque to build up in the arteries. The LDL stands for "low density lipoprotein." HDL stands for "high density lipoprotein." The low density cholesterol tends to stick, where as the high density moves right along. When the LDL is high you stand a risk of too much sticking - and the heart attack and stroke risks go way up.

The LDL harms the body if left untreated. Untreated the blood will quit carrying it and it will fall and stick to the walls of the arteries and blood vessels. This can cause clots and blockages that can block blood from reaching the brain or the heart, which will cause a stroke or heart attack and can kill a person. This is why it is so important to treat and prevent high cholesterol. The first line of defense in both treatment and prevention is in the diet.

A low cholesterol diet will encourage the good HDL cholesterol to be at a healthy level. This cholesterol actually scrubs the bad LDL from the artery walls, so you want this to be in the good normal range. Unfortunately,

LDL cholesterol is more abundant than HDL and could be even more so if a person does not eat right.

All cholesterol is vital to the body, it just needs to be there in optimal levels and not too high or too low. The liver naturally creates cholesterol. The issues come in because animals also create it naturally and if we consume these animals (like liver, dairy products, etc.) we will have that added on top of what our body normally manufacturers. If you look at the cholesterol in foods, if you can see the composition amount of the cholesterol, you would want to keep the consumption of it to 300 mg or lower a day. Unfortunately, again, the average American diet consists of much more than the recommended amount. This could be why there are more obese people in the USA and people with high cholesterol issues.

Consuming too much fat from the diet will cause the cholesterol levels to rise up too. Fat exists in animal products like dairy products, bacon grease, and in parts of what is otherwise lean meats like chicken skin. Consuming too much of these will cause the LDL levels to rise.
There are different types of fats in foods. Animal fat is called saturated fat. There are also unsaturated fats that are classified as either polyunsaturated or

monounsaturated. Both of these are good fats, but monounsaturated fats are the best, beneficial and in fact help to bring cholesterol levels down to normal readings. Monounsaturated fats are in canola oil, olive oil and peanut oil. Polyunsaturated fats, which are okay, are found in corn oil, safflower oil, soybean oil, and sunflower oil. Another polyunsaturated oil, which is very beneficial to the body, to the brain and in helping to strengthen the heart, is omega-3 fatty acid. This is found in most fish and in flax seeds.

The worst type of fat is trans fat which is a man made substance found in partially hydrogenated or hydrogenated vegetable oils. Trans fat reacts the same as saturated fat in the body and thus raises the LDL cholesterol levels. Trans fat was high in margarines years ago. Now, most margarine brands do not have it, but a few may. It pays to read the labels and find out.

No matter the reason for high blood cholesterol levels, they need to be reduced immediately. Diet and exercise are sometimes all it takes to lower the bad cholesterol levels. Physicians may give their patients anywhere from six to twelve weeks of good dieting and exercise to naturally lower their cholesterol levels, and if this does not work, they may have to prescribe medications. For many though, diet and exercise do help to reduce the numbers significantly so that prescription medications are not necessary.

Always read labels on all the foods you purchase especially if it is a prepared food. All labels should have this information: total fat including trans fat, saturated fat (and may list the mono and poly too), calories, carbohydrates, dietary fiber, plus the amount of sodium, sugar, and some of the vitamins and minerals like A, C and calcium and iron. Knowing the numbers will help you to choose the right foods to keep on your low cholesterol diet.

This book will help with the recipes, which are geared to include the healthiest foods out there. Diet and exercise go hand in hand, and this includes help to lower cholesterol in the body too. Make sure to discuss any new diet with your health care provider first.

Section 1: Superfoods

Before we say anything else about superfoods and the recipes that you'll find in this book, it's important to mention that superfoods isn't a term which nutritionists or dieticians use. In fact, there isn't any single, universally accepted definition of the term, although it is used to market all manner of food products and nutritional supplements. That doesn't mean, however, that some foods aren't, for lack of a better term, super in terms of their nutritional value and health benefits.

Perhaps the most useful definition of superfoods is this: a food which is rich in essential nutrients, phytochemicals and other beneficial compounds, but that is also healthy in the broadest sense. These are fairly low calorie foods which contain no additives or artificial ingredients.

The best superfoods are also some of the easiest to find at your local market. Foods like pumpkin and other winter squashes, wild salmon, beans and lentils, spinach and other dark leafy greens, blueberries, kiwi fruit, oats, sweet potatoes and even chocolate (dark chocolate, not milk chocolate). Common though these foods may be, they all meet the superfoods criteria and are highly nutritious, healthy foods which deserve a prominent place in anyone's diet.

We'll go into the nutritional benefits of these superfoods in a little more detail in the individual chapters which follow. From vitamins and to phytonutrients which may play a role in preventing illness, to fiber and of course, flavor, these are foods which have a lot to offer your palate and your health.

Salmon

Salmon is the exception among superfoods in that it's an animal product rather than a fruit, vegetable or seed. Salmon is one of the richest sources of omega-3 fatty acids, a compound which can promote cognitive development, possibly improve mood and fight inflammation (and as such, is thought to help prevent certain forms of cancer as well as stroke and heart disease, among other illnesses). It's also an excellent source of lean protein and vitamin D, as well as carotenoid compounds (which are what give salmon its distinctive color).

One important thing to keep in mind when you're choosing salmon at your local market is to always opt for wild caught salmon. Farmed salmon will do in a pinch, but studies have shown that farmed salmon tends to contain lower levels of omega 3 fatty acids as well as having levels of PCB and dioxins which are as much as eight times higher than those found in their wild caught counterparts – as with any other food, it seems that the more natural your salmon is, the better it is for you.

Sweet Coconut Crusted Salmon

Number of servings: 4

Ingredients:

4 salmon filets, about 4 ounces each
1 cup butter
¾ cups coconut flakes
¾ cup honey

Preparation:

Place the butter in a small saucepan over medium heat. Melt the butter, then mix in the coconut flakes and honey once the butter has melted completely. Stir well to combine and bring to a boil, then remove from heat. Allow the mixture to cool slightly, then transfer to a large bowl. Add the salmon, turn to coat the fish with the butter, honey and coconut mixture, cover and refrigerate. Allow to marinate for at least 30 minutes while you preheat your oven to 375 F.

Pour a little of the marinade into a baking dish; just enough to coat the bottom. Place the salmon filets in the dish and pour marinade over the top, reserving a little for basting. Transfer the dish into the oven and bake for 25 minutes or until the salmon flakes easily with a fork, basting occasionally with the remaining marinade. Remove from the oven and serve hot.

Salmon Quiche

Number of servings: varies (recipe yields 1 9" quiche)

Ingredients:

1 lb wild salmon, cooked, deboned and flaked
1 9" pre-made pie crust
4 ounces sharp cheddar cheese, cubed
4 ounces sharp cheddar cheese, shredded
4 eggs
½ of a small red onion, diced
½ cup milk
½ tsp dried sage
½ tsp dried parsley
½ tsp garlic powder
salt and black pepper, to taste

Preparation:

Start by preheating your oven to 375 F. Add the eggs, onion, milk and cubed sharp cheddar cheese to a blender or food processor, along with the spices and a little salt and black pepper. Blend until smooth. Place the crust into a 9" pie tin and spread with flaked salmon. Top with half of the shredded cheddar cheese, then pour the egg mixture over the salmon and cheese, then top with the remaining shredded cheese. Transfer to the oven and bake for about 30 minutes, or until a toothpick inserted into the center of the quiche comes out clean. Remove from the oven and allow the quiche to cool for 5 minutes before slicing and serving.

Quick and Easy Pan Fried Salmon

Number of servings: 2

Ingredients:

2 salmon filets (with skin), about 4 ounces each
2 tbsp olive oil
salt and black pepper, to taste

Preparation:

Rinse the salmon filets well and pat dry with paper towels until excess moisture is removed. Season the filets with a little salt and black pepper. Set aside.

Heat the olive oil over medium high heat in a heavy skillet. Once the oil is hot, place it gently into the skillet, skin side up. Cook for 5 – 7 minutes or until the flesh side is golden brown. Turn the filets over and cook for another 5 minutes, or until the skin side is lightly browned. Remove the salmon from the skillet and transfer to a plate covered with paper towels to drain off any excess oil. Transfer to individual plates and serve hot.

Tunisian Style Baked Salmon

Number of servings: 4

Ingredients:

4 salmon filets, about 4 ounces each
2 thin slices of red onion, separated into rings
4 thin lemon slices (slices, not wedges)
¼ cup mayonnaise
1 tbsp dry white wine
1 tsp fresh lemon juice
2 tsp harissa, or more to taste*
1 tsp paprika (use smoked paprika if you can get it)
1 tsp canola oil
salt and black pepper, to taste

* Harissa is a North African hot sauce made from chili peppers, caraway and other spices. If you don't have a middle eastern market in your city, you can make a close approximation of harissa by adding a little bit of crushed garlic and ground caraway seed to Rooster or a similar Thai chili sauce. If you can find harissa in your city, however, the real thing is definitely preferable.

Preparation:

Start by preheating your oven to 425 F and lightly oil a large baking dish with canola oil. Season the salmon filets with a little salt and black pepper and transfer to the baking dish. Top the filets with onion and a lemon slice each. In a small bowl, mix together the mayonnaise, harissa, lemon juice and paprika, then mix until thoroughly combined. Spread the mixture over the fish, lemon and onion, then drizzle the wine over the top.

Transfer the salmon to the oven and bake until it begins to turn opaque (about 10 minutes), then turn on your broiler and broil for about 3 minutes or until the fish is nicely browned on top. Remove from the oven and serve hot.

Baked Salmon with Lemon and Dill

Number of servings: 4

Ingredients:

4 salmon filets, about 4 ounces each
¼ cup melted butter
juice of ½ lemon
1 tbsp dried dill
2 tsp crushed garlic (about 2 cloves)
salt and black pepper, to taste
cooking spray

Preparation:

Preheat your oven to 350 F and lightly coat a baking dish with cooking spray. Place the salmon filets in the dish. Whisk together the melted butter and lemon juice and drizzle over the salmon, then top with the spices and a little salt and pepper. Transfer the salmon to the oven and bake for 25 minutes, or until the salmon easily flakes with a fork. Remove from the oven and serve at once.

Salmon Ceviche

Number of servings: 6

Ingredients:

1 lb high quality salmon filets, sliced thinly (use sushi-grade salmon if possible)
1 avocado, sliced thinly
1 tomato, diced small
2 cloves of garlic, minced
½ of a small red onion, minced
2 tbsp minced cilantro
¼ cup extra virgin olive oil
juice of 4 limes
2 tbsp salt
a pinch of cumin
a pinch of sugar
black pepper, to taste

Preparation:

Mix together the salt, sugar and lime juice in a large bowl, then stir in the cumin and black pepper. Add the remaining ingredients, gently mix to combine, cover and refrigerate for at least 4 hours or overnight to marinate.

Season to taste with black pepper before serving.

Salmon – Cream Cheese Dip

Number of servings: varies

Ingredients:

½ pound cooked salmon, skin and bones removed and flaked
8 ounces cream cheese, softened at room temperature
½ cup plain Greek yogurt
2 tbsp butter, softened at room temperature
2 tbsp diced pimentos
1 tbsp finely chopped Italian parsley
2 tsp minced red onion
1 tsp dill

Preparation:

Combine all of the ingredients in a bowl, except for the salmon. Blend until smooth with an electric mixer. Stir in the salmon, cover and refrigerate for a few hours or overnight.

Spinach

Spinach, like many other leafy greens, is one of those vegetables that many people hate as children and love as adults. Even if you don't think that you like spinach, the health benefits of this nutritional powerhouse alone merit another try – and when it's prepared as a part of delicious meals like these, you may well find that you like it after all!

Spinach is an excellent source of many vitamins, minerals and other nutrients, most notably vitamin C, vitamin K, folate, zinc and selenium, as well as smaller amounts of protein, vitamin E, magnesium, niacin and omega-3 fatty acids, among others. Popeye was on to something, certainly and so were your parents; they weren't trying to be mean to you by making you eat your spinach as a child. If any food deserves the title of superfood, spinach certainly fits the bill.

Spinach is wonderful cooked in a variety of dishes, but like any other vegetable, you'll get the most benefit by eating it raw or very lightly cooked. The following recipes include a few such dishes, but either way, don't skip (or skimp on) this ultranutritious leafy green!

Spinach, Lentil and Bean Curry

Number of servings: 4

Ingredients:

4 cups chopped fresh spinach, loosely packed
1 cup cooked kidney beans, drained and rinsed if using canned
1 cup dried red lentils
½ cup plain yogurt
2 medium sized tomatoes, diced
1 medium sized onion, diced
3 cloves of garlic, minced
1" piece of ginger, grated or crushed
¼ cup pureed tomatoes
2 tbsp chopped cilantro
2 tbsp canola oil
2 tsp garam masala
1 tsp turmeric
1 tsp cumin
1 tsp ancho chili powder
salt and black pepper, to taste

Preparation:

Rinse the lentils and place in a small saucepan with water to cover. Bring the lentils to a boil, then reduce heat to low, cover the saucepan and simmer for 20 minutes, or until the lentils are tender and have absorbed most of the water. Drain off any excess water and set aside.

Mix together the yogurt, tomato puree and spices in a bowl and combine well while heating the oil over medium heat in a large, heavy skillet. Add the garlic, ginger and onion and cook, stirring regularly until the onion starts to brown. Add the spinach and cook until just wilted, then stir in the yogurt mixture, cilantro and tomatoes. Add the cooked lentils and kidney beans, stir to combine and cook for 3 – 4 minutes or until the lentils and beans are heated through. Remove from heat and serve.

Beef Stew with Spinach

Number of servings: 6

Ingredients:

1 lb lean beef round, sliced thinly and cut into bite sized pieces
2 bunches of fresh spinach, rinsed well, patted dry and torn into 1" pieces
6 Roma tomatoes, diced
1 medium sized yellow onion, diced
4 small potatoes, quartered
4 cloves of garlic, minced
2 cups pureed tomato
1 ¾ cups beef broth
½ cup dry red wine
2 tbsp chopped fresh oregano
vegetable oil, for browning (about 1 tbsp)
salt and black pepper, to taste

Preparation:

Heat the vegetable oil in a skillet over medium high heat. Add the beef and cook until well browned, then transfer the beef to a stock pot. Add the onions and garlic to the skillet and cook in the remaining oil and fat until tender and lightly browned, stirring occasionally. Add the tomatoes and cook until about half of the liquid has evaporated, then transfer the mixture to the stock pot along with the beef.

Add the potatoes to the skillet and brown over medium high heat, turning occasionally to brown all sides. Transfer the potatoes to the stock pot, along with the spinach, pureed tomato, red wine, garlic and oregano. Add the beef broth, bring to a boil, then reduce the heat to a simmer, cover and cook for about 1 hour. Season to taste with salt and black pepper and serve.

Curried Spinach and Chickpeas

Number of servings: 4

Ingredients:

1can (15 ounces) chickpeas, drained and rinsed (or 1 ½ cups homemade)
2 large bunches of fresh spinach, washed, stems removed
1 package (12 ounces) firm tofu, cubed
1 medium sized yellow onion, diced
2 cloves of garlic, minced or crushed
1 tbsp curry paste (your choice)
1 tbsp canola oil
salt and black pepper, to taste

Preparation:

Heat the oil in a large skillet or wok over medium heat; once the oil is hot, add the onions and sauté until translucent, stirring regularly. Add the curry paste and garlic and cook for 3 minutes, stirring occasionally. Add the chickpeas and tofu and stir gently. Reduce the heat slightly and cover. Cook, covered for 2 – 3 minutes or until the spinach is just wilted. Remove from heat, season to taste with salt and black pepper and serve.

Wilted Spinach Salad with Goat Cheese and Cherries

Number of servings: 4

Ingredients:

1 bag (10 ounces) baby spinach leaves
1 small red onion (or ½ of a medium sized onion), diced
2 cloves of garlic, minced
1 cup sliced crimini mushrooms
¼ cup dried tart cherries
2 tbsp crumbled goat cheese
1 tbsp olive oil
black pepper, to taste

Preparation:

Heat the olive oil over low heat in a large skillet. Add the onion, garlic, mushrooms and cherries and cook, stirring regularly, for about 5 minutes, or until the mushrooms and onions are tender but not browned. Add the spinach and cook until just wilted, about 3 minutes. Remove from heat, divide among individual plates and serve topped with a little goat cheese and black pepper.

Baked Spinach and Feta Pitas

Number of servings: 6

Ingredients:

6 whole wheat pitas (6" size)
2 Roma tomatoes, diced
1 bunch spinach, washed, patted dry and chopped
4 crimini mushrooms, sliced
6 ounces sun dried tomato pesto
½ cup crumbled feta cheese
3 tbsp olive oil
black pepper, to taste

Preparation:

Preheat your oven to 350 F while you prepare your pitas for baking. Spread each piece of pita with sun dried tomato pesto and place on a large baking sheet, pesto side up. Top the pitas with spinach, tomatoes, mushrooms and feta. Drizzle with a little olive oil and a sprinkling of black pepper.

Transfer the baking sheet to the oven and bake for 10 – 12 minutes, or until the pitas are crisp and the toppings are slightly browned. Slice each pita into quarters and serve immediately.

Chicken Florentine

Number of servings: 4

Ingredients:

4 chicken breast halves, skinless, boneless and sliced
into strips
8 ounces penne pasta, uncooked
2 cups loosely packed spinach leaves
2 cloves of garlic, minced
4 tbsp pesto
2 tbsp olive oil
1 tbsp grated Romano or Parmesan cheese

Preparation:

Heat the oil over medium high heat in a large skillet
while bringing water to a boil to cook the pasta. Once
the oil is hot, add the garlic and sauté for about 1 minute
or until it becomes fragrant. Add the chicken breasts and
cook for 7 – 8 minutes per side. When the chicken is
close to being cooked through, add the spinach and cook
for 3 – 4 minutes, or until just wilted. Reduce the heat to
low.

Once the pasta is finished, drain and rinse under cold water. Return to the pan. Add the chicken mixture, then the pesto. Stir well to combine, divide among individual plates and serve, topped with a little Romano or Parmesan cheese.

Fruit and Spinach Smoothie

Number of servings: 2

Ingredients:

1 banana, cut in half
1 cup of frozen grapes
½ apple, cored and diced
1 ½ cups baby spinach leaves
2/3 cup plain Greek yogurt

Preparation:

Place all of the ingredients in a blender and blend until smooth, stopping to push down anything which sticks to the side of the blender. Transfer into glasses and serve.

Quinoa

Quinoa may be a relative newcomer to the North American diet, but it's been a staple in the cuisine of the Andes for millennia now. This plant, a relative of beets rather than an actual grain, is grown for its seeds, which closely resemble grains in taste and more or less play the same role as rice in many other cuisines. Quinoa provides a complete protein as well as being rich in magnesium, phosphorus, potassium and B vitamins.

Try quinoa in the place of rice or other grains, as a breakfast porridge, as a base for salads and anywhere else that your culinary creativity takes you – these recipes don't cover all the bases, but they make a great introduction to this versatile and highly nutritious seed.

Baked Quinoa Breakfast Cereal

Number of servings: 2 – 3

Ingredients:

1 cup quinoa
¼ cup flax seed
1 tbsp canola oil
2 tbsp maple syrup
1 tsp cinnamon
cooking spray

Preparation:

Preheat your oven to 350 F and lightly coat a baking sheet with cooking spray. Rinse the quinoa well and drain thoroughly (unless you're using quinoa which has been pre-rinsed), then add to a large bowl with the rest of the ingredients. Stir until well combined and spread out the mixture on the baking sheet, forming as thin of a layer as possible. Bake until golden brown, about 15 – 17 minutes, stirring every 5 minutes. Remove from the oven and allow it to cool completely before serving. This can be stored in a covered airtight container once it has cooled to room temperature.

Five Spice Quinoa

Number of servings: 4

Ingredients:

2 cups water
1 cup quinoa, rinsed and drained
1 beef bouillon cube
1 ½ tbsp butter
1 tbsp five spice powder
½ tsp powdered ginger
black pepper, to taste

Preparation:

Place all of the ingredients except for the quinoa in a saucepan and bring to a boil, stirring until the bouillon cube is dissolved. Add the quinoa, reduce the heat to a simmer, cover and cook for about 20 minutes or until the quinoa has absorbed all of the liquid and is tender.

Quinoa Pilaf

Number of servings: 4

Ingredients:

1 cup quinoa, rinsed and drained
1 small yellow onion, diced
2 medium sized carrots, diced
2 cups vegetable stock
¾ cup chopped walnuts
¼ cup chopped Italian parsley
1 tbsp olive oil
salt and black pepper, to taste

Preparation:

Heat the olive oil in a saucepan over medium high heat.
Once the oil is hot, add the onion and cook until
translucent, stirring occasionally. Add the carrots and
cook for another 3 minutes. Add the vegetable stock and
quinoa and bring the mixture to a boil. Reduce the heat
to a simmer, cover and cook for 15 – 20 minutes, or until
the quinoa has absorbed all of the liquid and is tender.
Transfer the cooked quinoa mixture to a bowl and toss
with the parsley and walnuts. Season to taste with salt

and black pepper; serve at once or allow to cool and serve at room temperature.

Quinoa and Mushrooms

Number of servings: 6

Ingredients:

1 ½ cups quinoa, rinsed
3 cups chicken broth
1 cup sliced crimini or button mushrooms
1 small yellow onion, diced
3 cloves of garlic, minced
1/3 cup grated Parmesan or Romano cheese
1 tbsp butter
1 tbsp olive oil
salt and black pepper, to taste

Preparation:

Heat the olive oil over medium heat in a large skillet. Add the mushrooms, garlic and onion to the hot oil and cook for about 5 minutes or until browned, stirring occasionally. Set aside.

Melt the butter in a saucepan over medium heat. Add the quinoa and brown, stirring regularly (this will take about 3 minutes). Add the chicken broth and bring the quinoa to a boil. Reduce the heat to low, cover and cook for about 15 minutes, or until the broth is almost absorbed. Add the mushroom mixture and cook for another 2 minutes, or until all of the broth is absorbed and the mushrooms are heated through. Season to taste with salt and black pepper, divide among individual plates and serve hot, topped with Parmesan or Romano cheese.

Broccoli and Quinoa Soup

Number of servings: 6

Ingredients:

2 cups of broccoli florets
2 cups chicken or vegetable broth
1 cup quinoa, rinsed
1 cup evaporated (not condensed) milk
½ of a medium sized yellow or white onion, diced
4 cloves of garlic, minced
1 tbsp flour
1 tbsp olive oil
salt and black pepper, to taste

Preparation:

Heat the olive oil over medium heat in a large skillet. Add the garlic and onion and cook until translucent, about 5 minutes, stirring regularly. Add the quinoa, broccoli and chicken or vegetable broth and bring to a boil. Cover, reduce the heat to low and simmer for 10 – 15 minutes, or until the quinoa is tender and fluffy and most of the liquid has been absorbed.

Add the flour and evaporated milk and bring the mixture back to a boil. Cook until the soup thickens, stirring constantly. Season to taste with salt and black pepper, divide among individual bowls and serve hot.

Quinoa Salad with Cranberries and Cilantro

Number of servings: 6

Ingredients:

1 cup quinoa, rinsed
1 ½ cups water
1 small red onion, diced small
¼ cup each diced red and yellow bell pepper
½ cup carrots, diced small
½ cup dried cranberries
¼ cup chopped cilantro
¼ cup toasted slivered almonds
1 ½ tsp curry powder (or more to taste)
juice of 1 lime
salt and black pepper, to taste

Preparation:

Bring the water to a boil in a covered saucepan. Add the quinoa, cover and reduce the heat to a summer. Cook for 15 – 20 minutes, or until the water has been absorbed and the quinoa is tender and fluffy. Transfer the cooked quinoa to a large mixing bowl and place in the refrigerator to chill. Once the quinoa is cold, stir in the remaining ingredients, season to taste with salt and black pepper and refrigerate before serving cold.

Beans and Lentils

Beans have something of a bad reputation due to their propensity to cause gas in many people, especially those who are unaccustomed to including them in their diet regularly. While there is no getting around this effect to some degree, beans are so nutritious that even this is no reason to avoid them entirely. When prepared properly and incorporated as a regular part of your diet, you'll find their less desirable effects greatly reduced and you'll enjoy their nutritional and health benefits in the bargain.

Beans and lentils are rich in protein, being perhaps the single best vegetarian source of this essential nutrient. They're also a natural choice for anyone trying to lose excess weight or maintain their weight, since they're a naturally high fiber food. As we all know, fiber plays an essential role in regulating digestion and appetite, since fiber helps you stay feeling full for longer, which curbs the urge to snack or to overeat at meals. They're also one of the best kinds of carbohydrates to include in your diet. Refined carbs may have earned their bad reputation, but natural carbohydrates like those found in beans, vegetables and fruit are the kind that you want to include in your diet.

Vegetarian Chili

Number of servings: 8

Ingredients:

1 can (15 ounces) each of black beans, chickpeas and kidney beans, drained and rinsed – or 1 ½ cups each of homemade cooked beans
1 ½ cups corn kernels (frozen and thawed or fresh cut from the cob)
1 medium sized yellow or white onion, diced
2 green bell peppers, diced
2 stalks of celery, diced
6 cloves of garlic, minced
2 – 3 jalapeno peppers, diced
3 large cans (10 ½ cups total) of crushed tomatoes
2 (4 ounce) cans of green chilies
1 tbsp olive oil
2 tbsp oregano
2 tbsp chili powder (your choice)
1 tbsp cumin
1 tbsp salt, or to taste
1 tbsp black pepper, or to taste
2 bay leaves

Preparation:

Heat the olive oil over medium heat in a stock pot. Once the oil is hot, add the onion, oregano, cumin, bay leaves and salt. Cook until the onion turns translucent, stirring regularly. Add the peppers, garlic, celery and green chilies and cook for 3 -4 minutes, stirring occasionally. Reduce the heat to low, cover and simmer the vegetables and spices for 5 minutes.

Add the tomatoes, chili powder, black pepper and beans. Bring the chili to a boil, then reduce the heat to low, cover and simmer for 45 minutes. Add the corn, stir and cook for another 5 minutes to heat through before serving.

Pasta Fagioli

Number of servings: 8

Ingredients:

1 (15 ounce) can cannellini beans or 1 ½ cups
homemade cannellini beans
1 (15 ounce) can navy beans or 1 ½ cups homemade
navy beans
1 lb ditalini
1 large yellow or white onion, diced
4 cloves of garlic, minced
1 large (28 ounce) can pureed tomato
5 ½ cups water
3 tbsp olive oil
1 tbsp dried parsley
2 tsp each dried oregano and basil
1/3 cup grated Romano or Parmesan cheese
salt and black pepper, to taste

Preparation:

Heat the olive oil in a large saucepan or stock pot over
medium heat and cook the onion until translucent,
stirring occasionally. Add the garlic and cook until

fragrant, about 2 minutes. Reduce the heat to medium low and add the remaining ingredients except for the ditalini and cheese. Simmer for 1 hour.

Bring lightly salted water to a boil in another large pot and cook the ditalini until al dente. Drain the pasta and stir it into the soup. Season to taste with salt and black pepper and serve hot.

Cuban Style Black Beans

Number of servings: 12

Ingredients:

2 cups dry black beans, soaked overnight
1 medium to large yellow onion, diced
1 green bell pepper, diced
6 cloves of garlic, chopped
½ cup dry white wine
¼ cup olive oil
2 tbsp white or apple cider vinegar
1 tbsp salt, or to taste
1 tbsp black pepper, or to taste
1 tbsp cumin
1 tbsp oregano
2 bay leaves

Preparation:

Add the black beans to a stock pot with enough water to cover plus 2". Add the onion, green pepper, garlic, salt, cumin, oregano and bay leaves. Bring to a boil, then reduce the heat to a simmer and cook, covered for 1 -2 hours, adding water as necessary to prevent the beans from drying out or burning. When the beans are nearly done, add the wine, oil and vinegar and stir well. Continue cooking uncovered until the alcohol cooks off, remove from heat and serve.

Black Bean Hummus

Number of servings: 8

Ingredients:

1 (15 ounce) can of black beans, drained and rinsed (or 1 ½ cups homemade)
2 cloves of garlic, minced
2 tbsp water
2 tbsp tahini
juice of 1 lemon
1 tsp cumin
½ tsp salt
¼ tsp cayenne pepper, or more to taste
¼ tsp paprika

Preparation:

Add the black beans, garlic, water, lemon juice, tahini, cumin, salt and cayenne pepper to a food processor. Blend until smooth, adding additional water as needed. Transfer to a bowl, sprinkle with paprika and serve at once or chill until ready to serve.

Southwestern Breakfast Platter

Number of servings: 2

Ingredients:

1 (15 ounce) can of black beans, drained and rinsed (or 1
½ cup homemade)
4 eggs, beaten
1 avocado, peeled, seeded and sliced
¼ cup salsa (your choice), or more to taste
2 tbsp olive oil
salt and black pepper, to taste

Preparation:

Heat the olive oil in a small skillet over medium heat.
Add the eggs and cook until set, about 3 minutes. While
the eggs are cooking, microwave the beans for about
minute or until hot. Divide the beans between two
bowls and top each with eggs, avocado slices and salsa.
Season to taste with salt and black pepper and serve
immediately.

Lentil Soup

Number of servings: 8

Ingredients:

1 ½ cups lentils, soaked, rinsed and drained
3 ½ cups crushed tomatoes
2 celery stalks, diced
2 cloves garlic, minced
1 large onion, diced
2 medium sized carrots, diced
1 sprig of Italian parsley, chopped
7 cups chicken or vegetable stock
¾ cup dry white wine
½ cup grated Romano or Parmesan cheese
2 tbsp olive oil
1 tsp paprika
2 bay leaves
salt and black pepper, to taste

Preparation:

Heat the oil in a stockpot and sauté the onions until they turn translucent. Add the garlic, carrots, celery and paprika and cook for 10 minutes, stirring occasionally.

Add the tomatoes, chicken or vegetable stock and bay leaves. Stir and add the wine, then bring to a boil. Reduce the heat to a simmer and cook, covered for 1 hour or until the lentils are tender. Season to taste with salt and black pepper and serve, topped with chopped parsley and Romano or Parmesan cheese.

Baked Chicken and Lentils

Number of servings: 6

Ingredients:

2 lbs chicken, bone-in
1 ¾ cups chicken or vegetable broth
1 ¼ cups tomato sauce or pureed tomato
¾ cup dried lentils
1 large onion, diced
1 small carrot, diced
4 cloves of garlic, minced
juice of ½ lemon
1 tbsp olive oil
1 tsp rosemary
1 tsp basil
salt and black pepper, to taste

Preparation:

Heat the olive oil over medium heat in a large, heavy skillet. Once the oil is hot, cook the chicken pieces for 5 minutes per side or until the juices run clear and the chicken is lightly browned on both sides. Remove from the skillet and set aside. Add the onion to the skillet and cook until tender, stirring occasionally, then add the garlic, carrots and sauté for another 5 minutes, stirring occasionally.

Add the lentils and broth and bring to a boil, then reduce to a simmer, cover and cook for about 20 minutes. Return the chicken to the skillet and cook for another 20 minutes, adding a little water if necessary. Add the tomato sauce, rosemary and basil and stir. Once the lentils are tender, add the lemon juice, stir well and serve hot.

Apples

Apples may not contain the nutritional cornucopia that some other fruits and vegetables have to offer, but there's a lot to recommend these sweet, crisp and almost universally loved fruits. Their high fiber content and antioxidant content make them a natural health food – and studies suggest that an apple a day really may keep the doctor away. The regular consumption of apples has been linked to a lower risk of colon, lung and prostate cancers, as well as helping to control cholesterol levels and assisting in weight loss.

While apples are usually thought of as an ingredient in desserts and indeed, there are some dessert recipes for apples in this book, they're also a good fit for savory dishes where their sweetness plays off of the flavors of other ingredients and as a component of salads. Apples are great eaten out of hand, but it's well worth experimenting with using them in your cooking.

Apple Soup

Number of servings: 4

Ingredients:

2 Granny Smith apples, peeled, cored and cubed
1 small russet potato, cubed (peeling optional)
2 shallots, minced
2 tsp grated or crushed ginger
3 ¾ cups chicken or vegetable stock
½ cup heavy cream
2 tbsp curry powder
1 tbsp butter
salt and black pepper, to taste
plain Greek yogurt, for garnish

Preparation:

Melt the butter in a large saucepan over medium heat.
Add the shallots and sauté until translucent. Add the
curry powder and ginger and cook for 1 minute, stirring
regularly. Add the apples, potato and chicken or
vegetable stock. Bring the soup to a simmer and cook
until the potato is tender. Remove from heat and allow
the soup to cool slightly before transferring to a blender.

Blend until smooth and return to the pan. Add the cream and season to taste with salt and black pepper. Cook for a few minutes to heat through. Divide among individual bowls and serve hot, garnished with a dollop of plain yogurt.

Brown Rice Salad with Fruit and Nuts

Number of servings: 6 - 8

2 cups cooked brown rice, cooled to room temperature
3/4 cup fresh or frozen peas (thaw first if using frozen)
1 apple, diced
1/4 cup dried cherries, chopped
1/3 cup walnuts, chopped
1 bunch of chives, chopped
The dressing:
2 cloves of garlic, minced
2 tbsp miso paste
2 tbsp toasted sesame seeds
2 tbsp canola oil
2 tbsp balsamic vinegar or red wine vinegar
1 tbsp honey

Preparation:

Combine all of the ingredients for the salad in a large
bowl. Whisk together the ingredients for the dressing.
Stir the dressing into the salad, mixing well to coat.
Garnish with chives and sesame seeds and refrigerate,
covered, overnight to allow the flavors to blend.

Braised Escarole

Number of servings: 4

Ingredients:

10 cups roughly chopped escarole
1 large apple (your choice), cored and cut into wedges
(peeling optional)
2 strips of bacon
salt and black pepper, to taste

Preparation:

Cook the bacon over medium heat in a large skillet until
crisp. Remove and place on paper towels to drain. Add
the apples and escarole to the skillet and toss to coat
with the bacon grease. Season with a little salt and black
pepper, reduce the heat to a simmer and cook, covered
for 8 – 10 minutes or until the escarole is dark green and
wilted. Serve hot topped with crumbled bacon and salt
and black pepper to taste.

Apple Coleslaw

Number of servings: 6

Ingredients:

4 cups shredded cabbage
1 cup shredded carrot
1 Granny Smith apple, cored and shredded
2 tbsp honey
2 tbsp mayonnaise
2 tsp white vinegar or apple cider vinegar
salt and black pepper, to taste

Preparation:

Mix the cabbage, carrot and apple in a bowl and toss to combine. In a separate small bowl, whisk together the mayonnaise, honey and vinegar. Pour over the salad, toss to coat, season to taste with salt and black pepper, toss again, cover and chill until you're ready to serve the coleslaw.

Apple Chutney

Number of servings: varies (recipe yields about 5 cups)

Ingredients:

15 tart apples - peeled, cored, and diced small
1 yellow onion, diced
3 small (1") pieces of fresh ginger, peeled
1 cup white wine or apple cider vinegar
½ cup brown sugar
1 tsp white pepper
1 tsp cinnamon
1 tsp cardamom
½ tsp nutmeg

Preparation:

Mix together all of the ingredients in a saucepan and bring to a boil. Reduce heat and simmer, covered for 30 minutes, uncovering and stirring occasionally, or until the apples are very tender, adding a little extra water as needed. Remove from heat, remove the ginger and transfer to a bowl. Cover and refrigerate until you're ready to serve your chutney.

Apple Turnovers

Number of servings: 8

Ingredients:

4 Granny Smith apples, cored and sliced (peeling optional)
4 cups water
1 cup brown sugar
2 tbsp lemon juice
2 tbsp butter
1 tbsp water
1 tsp corn starch
1 tsp cinnamon
1 package (17.25 ounces) frozen puff pastry sheets, thawed
The icing:
1 cup powdered sugar
1 tbsp milk
1 tsp vanilla extract

Preparation:

Add the lemon juice, water and sliced apples to a large bowl (the lemon juice will prevent the apples from browning). Melt the butter over medium heat in a large skillet. Once the butter is melted, drain the apples and transfer to the skillet. Cook for about 2 minutes, stirring regularly. Add the sugar and cinnamon and continue cooking for another 2 minutes, stirring occasionally. Mix the water and corn starch and add to the skillet. Mix well and cook until the sauce thickens, about 1 minute. Remove from heat and allow it to cool slightly.

While the filling cools, preheat your oven to 400 F. Unfold the pastry sheets and trim each into a square, then divide into 4 roughly equal squares. Spoon filling onto the center of each square, then fold over into a triangle shape, pressing the edges to seal. Place the turnovers on a baking sheet, leaving a little space in between. Bake for 25 minutes or until they're lightly browned and puffed up. Remove the turnovers from the oven and allow them to cool to room temperature. Make the glaze by mixing together the sugar, milk and vanilla extract, then drizzle over the turnovers before serving.

Apple Crisp

Number of servings: 12

Ingredients:

10 cups sliced apples
2 cups brown sugar
1 cup oats
½ cup water
½ cup melted butter
1 cup plus 1 tbsp all purpose flour
1 tsp cinnamon
¼ tsp baking soda
¼ tsp baking powder

Preparation:

Start by preheating your oven to 350 F. Arrange the sliced apples in a large (9" x 13") baking pan. Mix together 1 cup of the brown sugar, 1 tbsp flour and 1 tsp cinnamon, then sprinkle over the apples, then pour water evenly over the ingredients in the baking pan.

In a bowl, mix together the oats, the melted butter, baking soda, baking powder and the remaining flour and brown sugar. Layer the mixture evenly over the apples. Transfer the baking pan to the oven and bake for about 45 minutes or until the top is golden brown. Remove from the oven and allow the apple crisp to cool slightly before serving.

Yogurt

In ancient India, yogurt was referred to as the food of the gods; and medieval Persian tradition held that the longevity ascribed to the prophet Abraham by the Bible and the Qur'an was due to his regular consumption of yogurt. While yogurt may not be divine as such, it certainly is healthy, delicious and deserves a place in your diet.

Yogurt contains lactobacilli and/or acidophilus, helpful bacteria which can improve digestion; in fact, even people who are otherwise lactose intolerant can often eat yogurt and enjoy its nutritional benefits. Additionally, plain yogurt, especially Greek style yogurt, is a good source of protein and calcium. It has been suggested by some studies that eating low fat yogurt regularly can also help to promote weight loss. Just remember to steer clear of fruit flavored, sweetened yogurt – if you want fruit in your yogurt, add fresh fruit to some plain yogurt. It's even more delicious and you won't miss the added sugar at all!

Yogurt Pound Cake

Number of servings: varies (recipe yields 1 10" bundt pan)

Ingredients:

2 ¼ cups all purpose flour
1 cup plain Greek yogurt
1 cup margarine, softened at room temperature (butter may be substituted)
1 ½ cups white or turbinado sugar
3 eggs
½ tsp salt
½ tsp baking soda
juice of 1 lemon
cooking spray

Preparation:

Preheat your oven to 325 F. Lightly coat the inside of a 10" bundt pan with cooking spray, then flour. Sift the flour, salt and baking soda and set aside. Cream the margarine (or butter) and sugar in a bowl, then beat in the eggs, one at a time. Add the lemon juice, then add the wet ingredient mixture and yogurt to the flour mixture, stirring just until incorporated.

Pour the batter into your prepared bundt pan and bake for 1 hour, or until a toothpick inserted into the center comes out clean. Remove from the oven and allow the cake to cool in the pan for about 10 minutes, then turn the cake out onto a wire rack and cool to room temperature before serving.

Yogurt Rice

Number of servings: 8 (about 4 cups)

Ingredients:

1 cup jasmine rice
2 cups water
1 cup plain yogurt
¼ cup milk
1 dried red chili pepper or more to taste, broken into a few pieces
1 tbsp ghee (clarified butter)
1 tsp mustard seeds (preferably black mustard seeds)
1 tsp turmeric
½ tsp asafoetida
4 curry leaves (may be omitted if you can't find these)
salt, to taste

Preparation:

Cook the rice in 2 cups water until tender. Keep covered and set aside. In a small skillet, heat the ghee over medium heat and add the chili pepper. Cook for about 30 seconds, or until fragrant, then add the mustard seeds and cook for another 30 seconds or until they begin to pop. Remove from heat and add the curry leaves, asafetida and turmeric. Transfer the spices and ghee to a large bowl and whisk together with the yogurt and milk. Fold in the cooked rice and stir well to mix. Allow the rice to cool to room temperature, season to taste with salt and serve.

Beet and Yogurt Salad

Number of servings: 2

Ingredients:

2 cups plain yogurt
1 ½ cups cooked beets, peeled, sliced and cooled to
room temperature
2 tbsp chopped cilantro
1 tbsp canola oil
½ tsp black mustard seeds
½ tsp cumin seeds
salt and black pepper, to taste

Preparation:

Heat the oil over medium heat in a skillet; once the oil is
hot, add the mustard seeds and cook until they begin to
pop, about 30 seconds. Add the cumin seeds, cook for
another 30 seconds, then remove from heat.

Mix the yogurt and beets in a large bowl, then add the
mustard and cumin seeds. Season to taste with salt and
black pepper, stir, sprinkle with the chopped cilantro
and serve.

Yogurt Chicken

Number of servings: 4 – 6

Ingredients:

4 skinless, boneless chicken breasts
1 cup plain yogurt
1 cup seasoned bread crumbs
¼ cup butter
juice of 1 lemon
1 tbsp chopped Italian parsley
1 tsp garlic powder
salt and black pepper, to taste

Preparation:

Preheat your oven to 350 F. Add the yogurt to a small bowl and stir well until smooth, then add the lemon juice and stir again. Mix together the bread crumbs, garlic powder and a little salt and pepper in a shallow dish.

Place 1 pat of butter for each chicken breast in a 9" x 13" baking dish. Rinse the chicken and pat dry with paper towels. Dip each chicken breast in the yogurt mixture, then roll in the bread crumb mixture to coat lightly. Place the coated chicken breasts in the dish and top each with another pat of butter. Sprinkle with parsley and bake for 1 hour. Remove from the oven and allow the chicken to cool for at least 5 minutes before serving.

Yogurt Parfait with Blueberries

Number of servings: 2

Ingredients:

2 cups plain yogurt
4 graham crackers, crushed
1 cup fresh blueberries

Preparation:

Spoon half of the yogurt into the bottom of 2 parfait glasses. Layer half of the graham crackers on top of the yogurt, followed by half of the blueberries. Repeat the layering process and transfer the parfaits to the refrigerator to chill before serving.

Haydari

Number of servings: 8

Ingredients:

2 cups plain yogurt
5 cloves of garlic, crushed
a pinch of salt
4 tbsp fresh dill, chopped
1 bunch of Italian parsley, stems removed and chopped
mint leaves, for garnish (optional)

Preparation:

Place two layers of cheesecloth in a colander placed over a medium sized bowl. Place the yogurt in the colander and cover the colander with plastic wrap. Allow the yogurt to drain for 8 hours. Transfer the drained yogurt to a large bowl, then mix in the crushed garlic, salt, dill and parsley. Stir well to combine, then transfer into a serving dish. Chill briefly and serve cool, garnished with mint leaves if desired.

Eggplant and Yogurt Salad

Number of servings: 4

Ingredients:

1 medium sized eggplant, cubed
1 bunch of scallions, trimmed and sliced
½ of a small bunch of cilantro, stems removed and chopped finely
1 ½ cups plain yogurt
½ cup water
1 tsp smoked paprika
salt and black pepper, to taste

Preparation:

Add the eggplant and water to a saucepan over medium heat. Cook until the water is evaporated and the eggplant is very tender. Mash with a fork to eliminate any large pieces and allow the eggplant to cool to room temperature. When the eggplant is cool, transfer to a large bowl with the scallions, cilantro, smoked paprika and yogurt and mix well to combine. Season to taste with salt and black pepper, stir again, sprinkle with the chopped cilantro, cover and refrigerate to chill before serving – this salad can also be served at room temperature, if desired.

Yogurt Salad Dressing

Number of servings: varies (recipe yields about 1 cup)

Ingredients:

1 cup plain yogurt
2 tsp fresh lemon juice
1 tsp Dijon mustard
1 tsp chopped Italian parsley
1 teaspoon chopped fresh chives

Preparation:

Beat the lemon juice and yogurt together until smooth.
Add the mustard, chives and parsley, stir to mix well,
then cover and refrigerate until you're ready to use the
dressing.

Spinach Dip with Yogurt

Number of servings: varies (recipe yields about 3 cups)

Ingredients:

1 cup plain yogurt
1 cup fresh spinach, chopped
½ cup mayonnaise
2 tsp salt
1 tsp dried parsley
¼ tsp basil
¼ tsp oregano
¼ tsp dry mustard
¼ tsp garlic powder, or more to taste
black pepper, to taste

Preparation:

Mix together all of the ingredients in a medium sized bowl, stirring well to combine. Cover and chill until ready to serve.

Turkish-Style Zucchini Salad

Number of servings: 4

Ingredients:

2 zucchini, grated
2 cups plain yogurt
2 tablespoons chopped walnuts
2 tbsp olive oil
salt and black pepper, to taste

Preparation:

Heat the olive oil over high heat in a skillet. Add the zucchini and cook for about 3 minutes, stirring constantly. Remove from heat and allow the zucchini to cool to room temperature. Mix the cooled zucchini with the yogurt and walnuts and season to taste with salt and black pepper. Cover and refrigerate until ready to serve.

Sweet Potatoes

There is an interesting and little known fact about this ultra-nutritious member of the morning glory family (despite the name, they're not related to potatoes, nor are they the same as yams, which are an unrelated root vegetable commonly eaten in Africa and the Caribbean): they're the only food which provides all of the essential nutrients the human body needs. You literally could eat nothing but sweet potatoes and still meet all of your nutritional requirements – although you'd probably get sick of sweet potatoes pretty fast!

While it's not necessary to go on an all sweet potato diet, these starchy tubers are delicious and nutritious enough that they should show up at your dinner table regularly. They're an especially good source of vitamin A and beta carotene, but this is a vegetable which truly has a little bit of everything and is adaptable enough to be perfect in both savory and sweet dishes.

Sweet and Spicy Sweet Potatoes

Number of servings: 4

Ingredients:

2 large sweet potatoes, cubed (peeling optional)
3 tbsp olive oil
1 tbsp paprika
2 tsp brown sugar
1 tsp garlic powder
1 tsp onion powder
1 tsp poultry seasoning
½ tsp chili powder
½ tsp cayenne pepper, or more to taste
salt and black pepper, to taste

Preparation:

Start by preheating your oven to 425 F. In a large mixing
bowl, mix together all of the ingredients and toss to
coat. Spread the sweet potatoes in a single layer on a
baking sheet. Bake for 15 minutes, then turn and bake
for another 15 minutes or until tender and golden
brown.

Sweet Potato Soup

Number of servings: 8

Ingredients:

2 large sweet potatoes, peeled and cubed
1 medium sized yellow onion, sliced
2 cloves of garlic, sliced thin
1 Roma tomato, diced
4 cups chicken or vegetable stock
½ cup plain yogurt
¼ cup peanut butter
2 tbsp chopped cilantro
2 tbsp grated ginger
1 tbsp butter
1 tsp cumin
1 tsp crushed red pepper flakes
juice of 1 lime
zest of ½ lime
salt and black pepper, to taste

Preparation:

Mix the yogurt and lime zest in a bowl, then refrigerate.
Melt the butter in a large saucepan over medium heat.

Add the garlic and onion and cook until softened, stirring occasionally. Add the sweet potatoes and the chicken or vegetable stock, the cumin, ginger and crushed red pepper. Bring the mixture to a boil, then reduce to a simmer and cook, covered, for about 15 minutes or until the sweet potatoes are tender.

Transfer the soup to a blender and blend until smooth – you'll probably need to do this in batches. Return the pureed soup to the saucepan and whisk in the peanut butter and lime juice. Heat through, season to taste with salt and black pepper and serve hot garnished with diced tomato, chopped cilantro and a dollop of the yogurt and lime zest mixture.

Sweet Potato Rolls

Number of servings: 18 rolls

Ingredients:

3 ½ cups all purpose flour
½ cup pureed sweet potato
½ cup warm water
3 tbsp butter, softened at room temperature
2 tbsp sugar
2 eggs, lightly beaten
1 tsp salt
1 package active dry yeast

Preparation:

Dissolve the yeast and half of the sugar in warm water in a large mixing bowl; allow to stand for 5 minutes. Add the sweet potato, the rest of the sugar, the butter, salt and eggs and mix well. Add 3 cups of the flour, stir and turn out the dough onto a lightly floured work surface. Knead for a few minutes, adding a little extra flour as needed to prevent the dough from getting too sticky. Shape the dough into a ball and place in a lightly oiled bowl. Cover with a clean kitchen towel and set in a warm place to rise for at least 1 hour or until doubled in bulk.

Punch down the dough and allow it to rest for 2 -3 minutes before dividing into 18 roughly equally sized balls. Place on a lightly greased baking sheet, cover and allow the rolls to rise until they double in size; this is a good time to preheat your oven. Bake for 15 – 20 minutes, remove from the oven and serve warm.

Oven Roasted Sweet Potatoes

Number of servings: 6

Ingredients:

2 large sweet potatoes, cubed
2 medium sized sweet onions, diced into 1" pieces
¼ cup toasted sliced or slivered almonds
3 tbsp olive oil
2 tbsp amaretto (optional)
1 tsp thyme
salt and black pepper, to taste

Preparation:

Heat your oven to 425 F. Toss all of the ingredients except for the almonds in a baking dish to combine. Cover with foil and bake for 30 minutes. Uncover and bake for 10 minutes, then sprinkle with the almonds and bake for another 10 minutes. Remove from heat, season to taste with salt and black pepper and serve hot.

Sweet Potato Chili

Number of servings: 8

Ingredients:

½ lb lean ground beef
½ lb lean ground turkey
2 sweet potatoes, diced
1 small sweet onion, diced (about 2/3 – ¾ cup)
2 small celery stalks,diced
1 large can (28 ounces) diced tomatoes
1 ½ cups cooked or canned black beans, drained and
rinsed if using canned
1 cup tomato sauce or pureed tomato
1 cup fresh or frozen corn kernels (thaw first if using
frozen)
½ cup water
1 tsbp hot chili powder
1 tsp cumin
1 tsp each garlic powder and onion powder
½ tsp cinnamon
salt, black pepper and cayenne pepper, to taste

Preparation:

Place the tomatoes, tomato sauce, sweet potatoes, onion, celery, water and spices in a slow cooker set on high. Cook for 5 hours, stirring occasionally. Brown the ground beef and ground turkey in a skillet over medium high heat; drain off any excess fat. Add the cooked meat, beans and corn to the ingredients in the slow cooker and continue cooking for another 1 -2 hours to allow the flavors to combine. Season to taste with salt, black pepper and cayenne pepper and serve hot.

Sweet Potato Pie

Number of servings: varies (1 9" pie)

Ingredients:

1 9" unbaked pie crust, your choice
2 cups mashed sweet potatoes
¾ cup brown sugar
¾ cup milk
½ cup whipping cream
2 eggs, beaten
2 tbsp melted butter
1 tsp vanilla extract
1 tsp nutmeg
juice of 1 lemon

Preparation:

Start by preheating your oven to 375 F. Mix together the mashed sweet potatoes and melted butter in a large mixing bowl, then add the beaten eggs, brown sugar, milk, lemon juice, vanilla extract, whipping cream and nutmeg. Beat well until the mixture is smooth and then pour into the pie shell. Bake the pie for 50 – 60 minutes, or until a toothpick inserted into the center of the pie comes out clean. Serve warm or refrigerate and serve chilled.

Spicy Roasted Sweet Potatoes

Number of servings: 4

Ingredients:

4 sweet potatoes, cubed
6 tbsp olive oil
2 tsp cayenne pepper or more to taste
salt and black pepper, to taste

Preparation:

Preheat your oven to 375 F. Place all of the ingredients in a large resealable freezer bag and shake to coat. Transfer the coated sweet potatoes to a large baking dish and arrange in a single layer. Bake for about 1 hour or until the sweet potatoes are tender, stirring a few times during baking.

Sweet Potato Fries

Number of servings: 4

Ingredients:

2 large sweet potatoes, cut into French fry-size pieces
1 tbsp olive oil or more, if needed
2 tbsp fresh rosemary, minced
salt and black pepper, to taste

Preparation:

Preheat your oven to 425 F while you prepare the sweet potatoes. Toss all of the ingredients together in a large bowl to coat and arrange the fries in a single layer on a baking sheet. Bake until tender and slightly crisp on the outside, 25 to 30 minutes. Remove from the oven, season to taste with additional salt and black pepper, if needed and serve hot.

Kiwi Fruit

Native to China, the Kiwi fruit has a delicious sweet and tart flavor which most people love. They're an excellent source of fiber, vitamin C, vitamin K and vitamin B6, as well as several minerals and antioxidants – the skin contains the largest amount of antioxidants, unfortunately, since the fruit's fuzzy skin is simply discarded by many people.

Kiwi fruit is a natural fit for a fruit salad, smoothies or eaten out of hand as a snack or light breakfast. Try adding these unusual, yet delicious and very healthy fruits to your diet – you'll be glad that you did.

Kiwi Salsa

Number of servings: varies

Ingredients:

6 kiwis, peeled and diced
1 small sweet onion, diced
1 jalapeno pepper, diced
1 tbsp olive oil
1 tsp honey
½ tsp cumin
a pinch of chopped cilantro
juice of 2 limes
salt and black pepper, to taste

Preparation:

Mix together all of the ingredients in a bowl, except for the salt and pepper. Taste and season with salt and black pepper. Stir again, cover and allow the salsa to rest at room temperature for 1 hour. Refrigerate until ready to serve.

Spinach Salad with Kiwi and Strawberries

Number of servings: 6 – 8

Ingredients:

8 cups spinach, rinsed and torn into bite-size pieces
3 kiwis, peeled and sliced
8 strawberries, quartered
½ cup chopped walnuts
¼ cup canola oil
2 tbsp raspberry jam
2 tbsp raspberry vinegar

Preparation:

First, make your dressing by mixing together the vinegar, jam and oil in a small jar. Seal and shake vigorously to combine. Refrigerate until ready to use. In a large salad bowl, combine the remaining ingredients, then toss with the dressing and serve.

Kiwi Sandwiches

Number of servings: 8

Ingredients:

16 slices of whole grain bread
1 cup finely diced kiwi
1 cup cream cheese, softened at room temperature
zest of ½ lemon
2 tbsp honey

Preparation:

Mix the cream cheese, honey and lemon zest in a small bowl. Cover and refrigerate for 24 hours. Spread 2 tbsp of the cream cheese mixture on one slice of bread, then top with 2 tbsp of diced kiwi, then another slice of bread. Repeat this process to make all 8 sandwiches.

Kiwi Strawberry Smoothies

Number of servings: 2

Ingredients:

1 banana, halved
6 strawberries, quartered
1 kiwi, peeled and sliced
¾ cup pineapple juice
½ cup frozen yogurt

Preparation:

Place all of the ingredients in a blender and blend until smooth. Divide between 2 glasses and serve.

Fruit Pizza

Number of servings: varies (recipe makes 1 12" pizza)

Ingredients:

1 (18 ounce) package refrigerated sugar cookie dough
1 cup frozen whipped topping, thawed
1 banana, sliced
1 kiwi, sliced
½ cup sliced strawberries
½ cup crushed pineapple, drained

Preparation:

Preheat your oven to 350 F. Press the dough evenly into a 12" pizza pan and bake until golden brown, 15 – 20 minutes. Remove from the oven and allow the crust to cool to room temperature. Once the crust is cool, spread it with the whipped topping and sliced fruit. Refrigerate until ready to serve.

Blueberries

It's hard not to love blueberries. They have a taste which is uniquely their own and that almost everyone adores – but there's a lot more than taste to recommend these tart little berries. They're bursting with phytochemicals and antioxidants which are thought may help to combat cancer and other diseases and are also a source (albeit not a major source) of more than a dozen different vitamins and minerals.

Regular consumption of blueberries may also help to control cholesterol levels, reduce the risk of heart disease and possibly even help to improve memory. With all of these health benefits, it's no surprise that blueberries show up on any list of superfoods – and even if you aren't especially concerned about their nutritional value, their taste alone is enough to keep you coming back for more.

Blueberry Pie

Number of servings: varies (recipe makes 1 9" pie)

Ingredients:

4 cups fresh or frozen blueberries (thaw first if using frozen)
¾ cup sugar
2 tbsp corn starch
1 tbsp butter
½ tsp cinnamon
¼ tsp salt
1 9" inch double pie crust (premade or homemade)

Preparation:

Preheat your oven to 425 F. Mix together the corn starch, sugar, salt and cinnamon. Sprinkle this mixture over the blueberries. Line a 9" pie dish with one crust, pour in the blueberry mixture and dot the top with butter. Cut the other pie crust into ½" wide strips and make a lattice top. Crimp the edges with a fork. Bake for about 50 minutes, or until the crust of your pie is golden brown.

Blueberry Granita

Number of servings: 4

Ingredients:

2 ½ cups fresh blueberries
¾ cup water
½ cup sugar
juice of ½ lemon

Preparation:

Add the blueberries and sugar to a food processor and blend until smooth. Strain the mixture through a fine strainer, using a wooden spoon to press the mixture through while leaving as much of the seeds and skin behind as possible. Transfer the strained puree to a shallow glass tray and stir in the water and lemon juice. Place the tray in the freezer and freeze for about 4 hours, stirring once an hour. Scrape the granite from the tray and spoon into chilled small ice cream dishes for serving.

Blueberry Salsa

Number of servings: varies

Ingredients:

2 cups fresh blueberries, chopped roughly
1 cup fresh blueberries, whole
½ of a jalapeno pepper, minced (may use more or less to taste)
½ of a small red onion, diced
2 tbsp finely diced red bell pepper
juice of 2 limes
salt, to taste

Preparation:

Combine all of the ingredients in a bowl. Taste and season with salt, if desired. Cover and transfer to the refrigerator. Allow the salsa to chill for at least 2 hours before serving.

Blueberry Chicken

Number of servings: 4

Ingredients:

4 skinless, boneless chicken breast halves
2 cups fresh blueberries or frozen blueberries (thawed first)
½ cup white wine vinegar
2 tbsp Dijon mustard
2 tbsp orange marmalade
1 tbsp olive oil
salt and black pepper, to taste

Preparation:

Add the orange marmalade and Dijon mustard to a bowl. Stir well to combine. Heat oil over medium heat in a large, heavy skillet and cook the chicken for about 5 minutes per side, or until it's browned on the outside but still a little pink on the inside. Spread the marmalade and mustard mixture over the chicken add the blueberries and continue cooking until the chicken is completely cooked through, about 10 minutes, stirring frequently. The chicken is done when a meat thermometer inserted into the thickest part of a piece reads 165 F or higher. Transfer the cooked chicken to a serving plate.

Pour the vinegar into the skillet with the blueberries, season to taste with salt and black pepper. Cook until the sauce has been reduced by about 1/3. Pour the blueberry sauce over the chicken and serve.

Blueberry Walnut Salad

Number of servings: 6

Ingredients:

1 (10 ounce) package of mixed salad greens
2 cups fresh blueberries
½ cup raspberry vinaigrette (premade or homemade)
¼ cup roughly chopped walnuts
¼ cup crumbled feta cheese

Preparation:

Add the salad greens, walnuts, blueberries and salad dressing to a large bowl and toss to combine. Top the salad with crumbled feta and serve.

Dark Chocolate

Although chocolate isn't exactly a health food, at least in the form that we usually eat it, dark chocolate does have some health benefits which make it worthy of inclusion in this superfoods book. Cacao, the seeds which chocolate is made from, are rich in antioxidant compounds which prevent cell damage and inflammation – and these properties may make them useful in preventing certain cancers and other illnesses.

The healthiest way to eat chocolate is to have raw cacao, although this is generally too bitter for Western palates accustomed to chocolate which has been heavily sweetened. However, dark chocolate is the next best thing – you can still enjoy its health benefits by having it as an occasional treat instead of less healthy chocolate alternatives like milk and white chocolate.

Spicy Dark Chocolate Cookies

Number of servings: 36 cookies

Ingredients:

8 ounces semi-sweet chocolate, chopped
4 eggs
3 cups all-purpose flour
2 cups butter, softened at room temperature
2 cups brown sugar
1 ½ cups dark chocolate chips
1 cup white sugar
½ cup sifted cocoa powder
1 tbsp baking soda
1 tbsp water
1 tbsp vanilla extract
2 tsp minced chipotle peppers in adobo (may use more if you'd like spicier cookies)
1 tsp salt
a little powdered sugar, for coating the cookies before baking

Preparation:

Add the flour, salt and baking soda to a mixing bowl and

whisk together to combine. Set aside. Place the chocolate in a microwave safe bowl and melt; you can also use a double boiler to melt the chocolate, if you prefer. Let the chocolate cool a little bit before you proceed.

Beat the butter, brown and white sugar, chopped chipotle pepper and cocoa powder in a large bowl, mixing until the ingredients form a smooth mixture. Beat in the eggs one at a time. Add the water and vanilla extract to the mixture and stir well to combine. Next, add the melted chocolate, followed by the flour, salt and baking soda mixture and stir. Fold in the chocolate chips, then cover and place in the refrigerator for at least 1 hour to chill.

When you're ready to make the cookies, preheat your oven to 350 F and cover two large baking sheets with parchment paper. Roll small pieces of dough into balls, using your hands. You should end up with somewhere around three dozen cookies when all is said and done, but if you want to make larger cookies, feel free to do so.

Set the cookies on your parchment paper lined baking sheets, leaving at least 1" in between and preferably 2"; these cookies will spread out and flatten as they cook.

Bake for 12 – 15 minutes, remove from the oven and allow the cookies to cool for a few minutes, then transfer to wire racks to cool to room temperature. Store in an airtight sealed container.

Dark Chocolate Truffles

Number of servings: varies (recipe makes about 36 truffles)

Ingredients:

1 2/3 cups semi-sweet dark chocolate chips or finely chopped pieces
2/3 cups whipping cream (don't use light whipping cream for this recipe)
¼ cup finely chopped pistachios for coating the truffles.

Preparation:

Pour the whipping cream into a saucepan and bring to a boil, then immediately remove from heat. Add the chocolate chips or pieces and stir to melt the chocolate and incorporate both ingredients into a smooth mixture. Place the chocolate and whipping cream mixture in the refrigerator and allow it to cool and thicken for at least 15 minutes.

While the chocolate is cooling in the refrigerator, cover a baking sheet with parchment paper. Measure out a heaping teaspoon of the chocolate mixture for each truffle and place the baking sheet into the refrigerator to cool for another 20 minutes. Remove the truffles from the refrigerator, roll into balls by hand (you may want to lightly flour your hands to prevent excess sticking), then roll in the chopped pistachios to coat. Transfer the truffles into an airtight sealed container and refrigerate until you're ready to serve them.

Oats

Oats are a food that we should all be eating more of. They're high in fiber and can help to regulate cholesterol levels – and they're good for more than just porridge. Oats can be included in soups, breads and all manner of other foods; and they're so good for you that you just might find yourself looking for excuses to include them in other dishes once you've tried the oat recipes below.

Bannocks (Scottish Oat Cakes)

Number of servings: 2 – 4, depending on how large you make them

Ingredients:

2 cups rolled oats
1 cup all purpose flour, sifted (you can also use ½ cup whole wheat and ½ cup all purpose)
½ cup milk
½ cup butter, softened at room temperature
1 tbsp sugar
a pinch of salt
cooking spray

Start by preheating your oven to 375 F. Add the salt, sugar, flour and baking powder to a sifter and sift well to combine, into a large bowl. Add the oats and stir to mix, then cut the butter into the dry ingredients using two knives or a pastry cutter to form a pastry-like dough. Add the milk a little bit at a time, stirring constantly.

Flour a work surface and turn out the dough. Roll out the dough to about ½" thick. Divide the dough into two, three or four pieces (depending how large you want to make your bannocks), place on a baking sheet lightly coated with cooking spray and bake for about 15 minutes, or until the bannocks are lightly browned on top. Remove from the oven and serve warm or allow to cool to room temperature before serving.

Pumpkin

There's a lot more to pumpkins than Jack o' lanterns and pie (and actually, most canned pumpkin pie filling is made from butternut squash – all winter squash are pumpkins, technically speaking). Small pumpkins tend to be less watery and much easier to cook as well as sweeter, having a flavor very close to butternut or Hubbard squash.

Whether you use an actual orange pumpkin or another winter squash, these vegetables are excellent sources of vitamin A, beta carotene, vitamin C, omega-3 fatty acids, iron and B vitamins. Winter squash of all types are definitely superfoods in every sense of the word and as you'll see in these recipes, they're a perfect fit for dishes which are sweet, savory and everywhere in between.

New England Style Pumpkin Bread

Number of servings: varies (recipe yields 3 small loaves)

Ingredients:

3 cups all purpose flour
½ cup whole wheat flour
4 eggs
2 cups pureed pumpkin (canned or homemade)
2 cups white or turbinado sugar
1 cup canola oil
2/3 cup water
2 tsp baking soda
1 tsp salt
1 tsp each cinnamon, nutmeg and ground cloves
½ tsp powdered ginger

Preparation:

Start by preheating your oven to 350 F and prepare
three small loaf pans by lightly greasing and then
flouring them. Set aside. While your oven is preheating,
add the eggs, oil, sugar, water and pumpkin to a large
bowl and mix well to blend thoroughly.

Mix the rest of the dry ingredients in a bowl, whisking to combine. Add the dry ingredients to the wet ingredients and mix just until combined; pour the batter into your greased and floured loaf pans. Transfer the loaf pans to the oven and bake for about 50 minutes, or until a toothpick inserted into the center comes out clean.

Oatmeal with Pumpkin

Number of servings: 1

Ingredients:

½ cup rolled oats (or quick cooking oatmeal, if you want to save time)
1 cup milk or almond milk
¼ cup pureed pumpkin, canned or homemade
1 tsp honey, or more to taste
a pinch of cinnamon
a pinch of salt

Preparation:

Add all of the ingredients except for the honey to a small saucepan and bring to a boil, then reduce the heat to a simmer and cook until the oatmeal reaches your desired thickness, stirring regularly to prevent burning. Remove from heat, pour into a bowl and add 1 tsp honey or to taste.

Pumpkin Pasta

Number of servings: 6

Ingredients:

6 ounces uncooked very small pasta (your choice)
4 cups chicken or vegetable stock
1 medium sized yellow onion, diced
1 cup pumpkin, peeled, cubed and cooked (other winter
squash may be substituted if desired)
1 cup cooked turkey breast, cut into ½" pieces
2 tbsp olive oil or canola oil
1 tsp dried thyme
salt and black pepper, to taste
grated Romano cheese, for garnish

Preparation:

Pour the chicken or vegetable broth into a large
saucepan and bring to a slow boil over medium high
heat. In a large, heavy skillet, heat the olive oil over
medium heat. Saute the onion until tender, add the
thyme and then pour in about half of the stock
simmering in the saucepan.

Add the pasta to the skillet, stir and bring to a simmer. Add broth slowly, about half a cup at a time, stirring as you go and adding more once the broth is almost absorbed. Continue until the pasta is cooked to al dente texture, then add the butternut or acorn squash and cooked turkey. Stir well and add more broth, cooking until all of the ingredients are heated through, about 5 more minutes. Remove from heat, season to taste with salt and black pepper and serve hot garnished with a little grated Romano cheese.

Pumpkin Tacos or Tostadas

Number of servings: 12

Ingredients:

12 corn tortillas or tostada shells
2 cups of pumpkin, butternut squash or acorn squash
½ cup water
1 small red onion, diced
1 medium sized tomato, diced
2 tbsp canola oil or olive oil
1 tbsp cumin
1 tsp ancho chili powder
salt and black pepper, to taste
sliced avocado, chopped cilantro, salsa and lime wedges,
for serving

Preparation:

Heat the canola or olive oil over medium heat in a large
skillet or saucepan. Once the oil is hot, add the pumpkin
or squash and cook for about 3 minutes, stirring
occasionally. Add the stock and cumin, stir and continue
cooking until the pumpkin or squash is fork tender,
about 8 minutes. Season to taste with salt and black

pepper, stir and divide the pumpkin mixture among the tortillas or tostada shells and serve topped with avocado slices and cilantro, with lime wedges and your choice of salsa on the side.

Superfoods Conclusion

You don't have to be a nutritionist to understand how much eating the superfoods featured in this book can benefit your health – and as you've already found out if you've been preparing these recipes, you don't have to be some kind of joyless health nut to enjoy eating them either!

Superfoods are all around us and you probably eat many of these foods already. Getting the most out of these foods is a matter of making a conscious decision to make them regular parts of your diet and of course, to try eating them raw when possible. Obviously, you're not going to want to eat raw quinoa, sweet potato or pumpkin, but don't overcook your food and you'll find that it tastes better as well as being healthier.

Eating superfoods should be part of a healthier lifestyle which includes a healthy diet and regular exercise. These healthy lifestyle habits work together to help you get the maximum nutrition that these foods offer and help you achieve better health and youthful energy which can last a lifetime.

Section 2: Gluten Free Cookbook

Gluten Free diets are typically entered into by necessity, not by chance. That doesn't mean, however, that there are no real benefits to making the choice to go gluten free. In fact, for those who are considering a diet that may help to lower their cholesterol and make other positive, long-term health changes, going gluten free has some potential health benefits that may not have been considered.

Going gluten free has become a fairly popular new trend. You might even consider it to be one of those diet "fads" that hit the magazine and book shelves every few years. The difference is that most fads are not healthy and really don't help a great deal. This fad--which is not really a fad--is being seen to increase the energy and to improve the overall good health of many people who use it.

Celebrities such as Gwyneth Paltrow and Chelsea Clinton are finding that gluten free works for them, and it can work for you too. It's quite likely that you're seeing more and more gluten free products hitting the supermarket shelves recently. For those who have no food allergies and aren't concerned with gluten in their diet, going gluten free is something you probably haven't explored very carefully. The reason for the growing number of gluten free foods is that many people have explored gluten free and found that even if they don't' have to utilize the diet, it's much healthier--quite like the paleo diets which are so popular.

What is Gluten?

Gluten is a kind of protein that is part of grains and cereal products such as wheat. It tends To make bread and foods elastic, or chewy tasting. It keeps food from being "sticky." Gluten is found in flour products of wheat, but more, it is also found in other grains.

There are such a wide range of people who have a problem with gluten that it is considered to be one of the big 8 which are mandated to be listed on food packaging. If you have a gluten intolerance or allergy, going gluten free for you isn't a choice, it's a necessity and you need To make sure that you don't accidentally take in gluten in some form by mistake.

Become an expert at reading the packaging and finding out precisely what is in the product and not just that, what it has come into contact with so that you know your products are gluten free.

People who have certain food allergies or disease processes such as Celiac disease may not be able to tolerate even a tiny amount of gluten in their diet. One of the most common questions to be found among those who are newly diagnosed with Celiac is what they can and cannot eat. Take that a step further and realize that not only edible products have gluten, but many inedible ones do as well. Be very careful to wash your hands after using some soaps, lotions and even pet foods as these have nominal amounts of gluten in them which could be transferred to your food if you don't wash carefully after using them.

Advantages of Going Gluten Free

Doctors and naturalists have taken a good look at gluten free diets recently and found that gluten free can help to improve the overall good health of even those who are not suffering from a gluten allergy.

It can help to improve your serum cholesterol level, may

also promote better digestion, and might even increase your energy, particularly if you may be suffering from a gluten allergy or intolerance. The reason for this is not that gluten itself is particularly unhealthy. Many of the foods which are made from gluten or with gluten incorporated into them tend to be less healthy than those which do not contain it.

Gluten Free Cooking

Gluten free foods impose some big challenges. It makes it hard to enjoy foods that you may have eaten your entire life, but with a little work, you can make those recipes your own and in many cases, you'll be surprised at what foods are out there are naturally gluten free.

For example, a vanilla milkshake made with all natural ice cream is normally gluten free. Fresh strawberries, spinach, fruits of nearly all types and vegetables are gluten free naturally.

Even many of your favorite snack foods will be gluten free. Potato chips and most corn chips which are fried or baked in corn oil or soybean oil are gluten free. Check the packaging, but most are baked or fried using heart healthy methods and so are gluten free without any help from you. While these are not the ideal snacks, they are able to be eaten in moderation.

While it may be moderately frustrating at first trying to replace things like cake flour and find ways To make pasta and cookies, the more you look at gluten free meals, the more you'll find that you can create nearly any recipe that you like with gluten free foods and emulate most any recipe that you'll find with common sense and a bit of skill in substitution.

Take a look your new diet and approach it with the attitude of exploring new things, a challenge rather than a chore and you'll find that in no time, you and your family have really conquered the world of gluten free cooking. You may even find that you enjoy cooking more and that eating is more fun, better tasting, and healthier by far than those which incorporate the very sticky gluten filled processed foods that you were accustomed to.

Which Foods Would Be Eliminated in a Gluten Free Diet?

In many cases, the foods which are not healthy for you anyway, particularly processed foods would be missing from your diet. Foods such as white bread, white crackers and other processed wheat products are going to be eliminated from your diet. Noodles of many types are foods which won't be allowed to be eaten, but they can be replaced with rice noodles and other forms of pasta which are healthy and tasty.

The problem is that many people like the taste of these foods, and don't consider the many unhealthy components that are part of them. Foods which are processed such as supermarket breads and pastries contain not just gluten, but unhealthy fats, many preservatives, and other chemicals that are higher in disease promoting ingredients.

What Makes Gluten Free a Good Choice?

Studies show that eating a low gluten or gluten free diet can lower your risk of some disease processes such as heart disease, certain types of cancer, type 2 diabetes, and many other long term health conditions. Your diet would be richer in fruits and vegetables and would quite likely contain many more foods that offer positive health benefits and a higher level of vitamins, phytonutrients, and antioxidants.

Making Gluten-Free Work for You

Every year more and more people are diagnosed with celiac disease. They are required to eat a gluten free diet. You perhaps are not required to go gluten free, but the health benefits of doing so are nothing short of amazing. Even if you do not have celiac disease or an allergy to gluten which compels you to avoid oats, wheat, rye and malt, if you follow the gluten free diet even loosely, you may find that you feel better, that your skin is much clearer, and that you may have a lower incidence of heartburn, fatigue, and cramping.

The poor vitamin absorption that takes place in Celiac disease can make the person who suffers from this disease feel very unwell, have side effects of loose stool and even depression. It is imperative to stay within the dietary restrictions which have been given to you and to understand why you have those restrictions.

Basing your diet on a gluten free approach may be a good idea, but for the Celiac sufferer, it's something that is non-optional. The very strict limitations that apply to the celiac sufferer would not apply to those who are making a choice to go gluten-free, but sticking as closely as you can to the gluten-free approach will improve your health by removing most of the high fats and fried foods that we should quite likely be avoiding anyway. It can be a genuinely healthy way to eat, improving your serum cholesterol and your energy. It's not necessary to be as strict with yourself, such as avoiding malt flavors, when you are not genuinely restricted, but staying close to the diet so far as main meal ingredients will be beneficial for your entire family.

Gluten Intolerance and Allergies

Today for whatever reason, many people are actively allergic to gluten, to wheat and to other components of wheat. The numbers of these people grow continuously every year. It is particularly difficult in the case of children to limit gluten in the diet. If their allergic reaction is bad enough, the reaction can be devastating and foods which have gluten must be completely eliminated. Using rice noodles and gluten free foods is an imperative, not a choice. In addition, some diseases exist which require that people who suffer from them do not have gluten of any type as part of their diet. This means that not only wheat, but other foods which contain gluten must be eliminated from the diet.

Celiac is a serious illness with real consequences if the sufferer does not eliminate gluten. Keep in mind that making the choice to go gluten free means that you can be a little more lenient with yourself. You may eat foods such as soy sauce and other things that are not available to the sufferer of celiac or gluten intolerance. To that end, our book contains only recipes that are strictly and completely gluten free in order to be useful to the user who has chosen to go gluten free, as well as to the celiac client, who has a need to follow a strict gluten free method of eating.

What Are You Giving Up?

One of the first comments that people make when considering a gluten free diet is that they won't be able to enjoy desserts and other things that they are accustomed to and simply want on an occasional basis. The fact is that some things will be off limits, specifically processed pastries and that type of foods. That doesn't mean that there is nothing to replace it.

Eliminating gluten from your diet does not mean sacrificing taste. In fact, quite the opposite. Many of the things that you eat on a gluten free diet will be sweet treats that you make yourself. They won't incorporate high fat and gluten, of course, but they will incorporate fresh fruits, even cocoa in some cases, so you won't lose your chocolate or some of the other foods that you love. They can be eaten sparingly and when created with the correct ingredients don't add gluten or even a high amount of empty calories to your meals.

Gluten Free foods don't have to be lacking in taste or fiber. Here are some wonderful examples of what can be done with gluten free cooking, listed for you in sections.

Main Dish Gluten Free Recipes.

Main dish recipes are one of the most difficult to accomplish without any gluten but with a little imagination and creativity, you can come up with some wonderful meals that are gluten free and have incredible taste and appeal. Some perfect examples of gluten free main dish recipes include these, which are all created for the person who really has to have no gluten at all incorporated into their diet.

Lamb with Yams and Apples

This is completely gluten free and offers great taste as well as ample nutrition. The pairing of apples and yams offers a little sweetness to the pork as well as keeping it moist.

You will need:

- 1/4 cup dark brown sugar
- 5 tablespoons butter, melted
- 1 tsp vinegar
- 1 tsp salt
- 1/2 tsp granulated garlic

- 2 apples, cored and sliced
- 2 sweet potatoes, peeled and sliced
- 2 chops, preferably the tenderloin style

To make:

Preheat oven to 400 degrees Fahrenheit.

Mix the sugar, the butter the vinegar and the spices.

Keep about a tablespoon of the butter mix and set it aside.

Add the apple and sweet potato to your brown sugar mix and coat them.

Place the apples and potatoes in a roasting pan and cover with foil. Bake for twenty minutes.

Meanwhile lightly brown the lamb in the remaining butter mix.

Remove the potato and apple mixture from the oven and add the lamb over the top of the mix.

Replace the dish in the oven and bake it for approximately 40 minutes until a meat thermometer shows that the lamb is cooked.

Cheesy Mexican Chicken

Cheesy chicken becomes an instant favorite when you create it combined with cheese. Low in fat and high in nutrients, chicken is a favorite food for about half the world. This has a bit of a bite to it, with the chili peppers and tomato added

You will need:

- 2 tablespoon of olive oil
- 1 can diced tomatoes
- 1/2 teaspoon sea salt
- fresh ground pepper
- 1/2 cup finely chopped green onion
- 1 chopped clove of garlic
- 1 tsp chopped fresh cilantro
- 1 can diced green chilies
- 1 can black beans
- 1/3 cup Colby jack cheese
- 2 cups cooked white rice

To make:

Chop the chicken into cubes and brown in the olive oil, sprinkling with the sea salt and pepper.

Add the remaining ingredients, excluding the cheese.

Allow to cook on the stove top on low heat for approximately 40 minutes, until chicken is thoroughly cooked and tender.

Serve over white rice, topped with shredded Colby jack cheese.

Broiled Steak Salad

Broiled steak offers a chance for a great deal of the fat from the meat to leak into the broiler tray below, while not using the grilling that has been shown to cause some health considerations. Broiling meat and adding it to the wide array of greens and fresh vegetables ends up with a healthy and delicious meal that is gluten free and oh-so delicious.

You will need:

- 4 tablespoons of olive oil
- 6 teaspoons of apple cider vinegar
- 1 teaspoon fresh cilantro, chopped
- 2 tablespoons of fresh parsley, finely chopped
- 1 bell pepper sliced in strips
- 3 finely chopped green onions
- 1 clove garlic, minced
- 2 Roma or other meaty tomato, diced
- salt and pepper to taste.
- 2 cups romaine lettuce
- 2 cups iceberg lettuce
- 2 cups baby spinach
- 1/2 cup raw mushrooms
- 1/4 cup part skim mozzarella cheese
- 2 sirloin or Delmonico steaks

To make:

Take one quarter of the garlic, and rub steaks.

Salt and pepper steaks to taste, and place below the broiler.

Allow steaks to broil turning once until cooked to your taste.

Tear greens, mix and set aside.

Combine remaining ingredients and set aside.

Remove steaks from the broiler and cut into strips about half an inch wide

Place greens into salad plates and top with strips of the steak.

Sprinkle with grated mozzarella

Drizzle the vegetable dressing over the steak and the salad greens till coated. Serve warm.

Hearty Steak and Cheese Soup

Steak soup is a hearty way to end the day and perfect for those cooler autumn or winter days. If you're ready for a warm ending to the day, you can add the veggies and meats to your crock pot and leave on low heat for about 6 hours and your soup will be ready for you when you arrive home after work.

Fresh raw vegetables are the best that you can get and will give your soup a wonderful flavor, but in the event that your raw veggies are off season, frozen vegetables will work nearly as well and most of the time does not cause the nutrients to erode. If you're really hungry, consider adding some canned or dried beans to your soup To make it a bit more hearty and rib-sticking.

You will need:

- 2 lbs. stew meat or diced steak
- 2 quart cans of tomato juice
- 2 cups beef broth
- 1/4 cup frozen corn
- 1/3 cup chopped green onion
- 1/3 cup chopped celery hearts
- 1 cup halved baby carrots
- 1 cup diced potatoes

- 1 cup tomatoes diced
- 1 cup whole green beans-raw
- 2 tsp. Sea salt
- freshly ground black pepper
- 1 clove garlic-finely chopped
- 1/2 cup chopped green pepper
- 1 cup shredded cheddar or Colby Jack cheese to top the soup.

To make:

Into 1 qt. of water put beef and boil for 1 hour on medium heat.

For a hearty, substantial soup, cut up the meat in small pieces and add salt and pepper to taste.

Add tomatoes, tomato juice, onions and celery. Also add other vegetables, such as diced potatoes, carrots, string beans, corn, peas, cabbage or chopped peppers.

Boil until all vegetables are tender.

Serve topped with shredded cheddar and then broil it for just a moment To make the cheese bubbly.

Beef and Broccoli

One of the favorite Chinese foods which can be created is the beef and broccoli that we all eat on our forays out to the Chinese restaurant. This recipe can be made gluten free and also a bit healthier by the removal of a few things and the addition of another set. Keeping your foods heart healthy as well as gluten free means not using some of the traditional Chinese food inclusions such as monosodium glutamate, but in many cases, with the right spices, you're not even going to miss it.

It typically comes as a surprise to people that soy sauce is not gluten free traditionally. Soy sauce does tend to have wheat in it, but you can get around that with several brands of soy sauce that are fermented naturally and do not include gluten. The gluten free soy sauce has the same great taste that you'd come to expect. While we did name a brand that we know to be gluten free, bear in mind that there are others and this is simply a guideline.

You will need:

1 pound lean beef, sliced thinly into bite-sized pieces.

Marinade for Beef:

- 1 egg
- 1/3 tsp salt
- 1 Tbsp stock
- 1 Tbsp cornstarch (corn flour)
- 2 Tbsp water

Remaining ingredients:

- 1 1/2 Tbsp sunflower oil
- 1 16 ounce bag of broccoli,
- 1 cup sunflower oil
- 2 Tbsp Kikkoman Gluten-Free Soy Sauce
- 1 Tbsp sugar
- a few drops of sesame oil
- 2 cloves garlic, crushed
- 1/2 cup chicken broth
- 2 Tbsp cornstarch

To make:

Slice your beef into tiny pieces and add it to the marinade. Marinate the beef for at least half hour before adding the 1 1/2 tablespoons of oil to beef, mixing it all in and marinating your beef for another half hour.

While the beef is getting ready in the marinade, you'll be using that time to prepare the vegetables.

Heat a wok or a heavy pot and add 1 cup of oil. Stir fry the beef and remove it, setting it aside on another plate. Drain the oil and wipe it clean of oil. Add one half cup of water to your pot and bring it to a boil, adding the broccoli to it. Cover and cook the broccoli after coming to a boil for about 5 minutes. Drain and remove the broccoli.

Heat the pan or wok with about 2 tablespoons of oil. Add the garlic and fry lightly. Add the veggies, the beef and mix them thoroughly. In the center of the pan, make a well of sorts and add all of the ingredients for the sauce. Stir the cornstarch into a tablespoon of water and use this to thicken your broth. Mix the sauce together with the other ingredients and serve hot accompanied by rice if you like.

Curried Chicken and Mango Summer Salad

Not only gorgeous because of the color, it's light and easy to accomplish for a summer meal. The main things which require any cooking are the chicken which can easily be broiled or grilled, keeping the kitchen heat to a minimum. Adding the mango to the meal makes it colorful and pretty, as well as lowering the calories and adding some phytonutrients. The yogurt adds a good dose of probiotics to your meal and all in all, this is one of the more healthy summertime quick meals you're going to find.

You will need:

- 3/4 cup plain Greek yogurt
- Juice of one half lime
- 2 teaspoons clover honey
- 1 teaspoon curry
- 1/8 teaspoon sea salt
- 1/8 teaspoon freshly ground pepper
- 2 cups cooked broiled chicken, cut into bite sized pieces
- 1 cup mango peeled and cubed
- About 10 leaves of Romaine lettuce

To make the salad:

Combine the first six ingredients in the list into a small bowl and stir it all really well.
Add the chicken and mango pieces and toss to coat.

On a salad plate, layer several leaves of crunchy Romaine.

Spoon the mango chicken mixture onto the top of the lettuce leaves and add a few pieces of chopped celery or cucumber for pretty and for crunch.

This delicious summer salad is also low in fat, low in calories and incorporates all of the health benefits that yogurt and mango have to offer.

Health Challenges in Our World

In the world today, some of the biggest challenges to our health include heart disease, stroke, Alzheimer's, cancer, and type 2 diabetes. Many of these things can be warded off if our diet becomes healthier and a little more natural. That means removing high fat foods, some of which are also high in gluten and replacing those foods with more natural foods such as fruits, vegetables and flour which is made of healthier ingredients. Whole grain foods are healthy in and of themselves, but once processed, contain additives which can be cancer-causing and high in fat.

Eliminating some of those foods can help To make a very positive change in your lifestyle and in your health. It may promote long term weight loss and change your life for the better. Adding more raw vegetables and even cooked or steamed will add further benefits to your long term good health.

Side Dishes and Vegetables

Vegetables are a very healthy part of your diet. So far as possible eating your vegetables raw is usually preferable in order to keep the nutrients sound. Many of the vitamins and minerals do not stay well during cooking or storage, with some being very unstable.

While there are exceptions to this rule, which will be named later, for the most part, keeping your vegetables raw will keep them more nutritious. Side dishes and salads are a very healthy part of your diet, combating some kinds of cancer as well as adding phytonutrients to your diet.

Winter Squash in Brown Butter and Parsley

Since this side-dish is prepared on the stovetop, it is especially nice for Thanksgiving and Christmas, when oven space always seems to be limited.

You will need:

- 1 ½ pounds winter squash, peeled, seeded, and cut into ½ inch cubes. (Acorn, or Butternut squash work well.)
- 4 Tbsp real butter
- 1 ½ Tbsp chopped, fresh parsley
- ¼ tsp salt
- ¼ tsp freshly ground black pepper
- 1 Tbsp brown sugar (optional)

To make:

Place butter in a large skillet over medium heat, stirring frequently with a whisk.

Once melted, the butter will foam a little, subside, milk solids will form and become a honey brown color. At this time the butter will have a strong nutty smell. (It take just a few seconds for your browned butter to burn, if this happens, you'll need to start over.)

Once the butter is browned, remove pan from heat and stir in fresh parsley.

Add cubed squash to pan, and turn to coat pieces evenly with butter, return to medium heat.

Allow the squash to cook on on side until it is lightly browned. This usually takes a few minutes. Continue turning squash to evenly brown all sides.

Reduce heat to low, and cover. Let squash cook until fork tender, around ten minutes.

Add brown sugar, if desired, just before squash is done, and turn to distribute evenly.

Chinese Green Beans

We all love those delicious green beans that we get in the Chinese restaurant. The secret is the sesame oil in many cases, and you can make the same thing at home in a really short time. Using gluten free soy sauce, sesame oil and a few other ingredients, you can get all the taste that you want and absolutely none of the gluten that might be found in a restaurant offering. Try out this recipe for Chinese green beans and you may never have to find them at the restaurant again.

You will need:

- 1 pkg frozen green beans , one pound
- 1 tablespoon gluten free soy sauce
- 1 can gluten free chicken broth
- 1 bunch green onions, about six
- 2 cloves of garlic
- 1/4 tsp ground ginger
- 1 tsp sugar
- 1 tbsp sesame oil

To make:

In a 2-quart casserole dish, combine green beans and broth. Cover and microwave 4 minutes on high. Make sure that your dish is microwave safe and remove it with an oven mitt.

Meanwhile, chop the onion and mince garlic.

Into a small bowl, put the ginger, soy sauce and sugar.

Add scallion rings and garlic. Set aside. Remove green beans from microwave and uncover.

Pour sauce over beans and stir.

Add to the microwave again for approximately 3 minutes. Remove and ensure they are heated through. Stir in the sesame oil and serve immediately.

High Energy Breakfast Smoothie

Smoothies or breakfast shakes can be a very healthy way to start your day when you're in a hurry, as we all are in the morning. Getting a good dose of veggies and fruits in a way that everyone can enjoy means that you start your day with a good breakfast, avoid all the gluten, not to mention the sugar, that you're going to get from a normal wheat-laden breakfast and you'll have the energy you need to face the morning.

You will need:

- One medium sized banana
- 1 slice fresh pineapple
- 1/4 cup fresh blueberries
- 1/4 cup sliced strawberries
- 1 cup skim milk
- 1 tablespoon honey

To make:

Simply combine all ingredients and blend till smooth in a high speed blender.

Heart Healthy Spinach Side Salad

Salad is a very healthy side dish and is almost always gluten free, depending on the dressing that you get. This side salad features some very heart healthy additions and also greens which have been chosen for their nutritional phytonutrients. Additionally the presence of lycopene in the tomatoes as well as the Omega fatty acids which are found in the sunflower seeds offers you a real boost to your health.

You will need:

-
  2 Roma tomatoes-quartered in wedges
- 2 cups Romaine lettuce
- 2 cups baby spinach leaves
- 2 cups iceberg lettuce
- 2 chopped green onions
- 1 cucumber, sliced in thin slices
- 2 tablespoons sunflower seeds

For the dressing:

- One quarter cup olive oil
- One quarter cup red wine vinegar
- 1 clove garlic, finely chopped

- 1 teaspoon cilantro chopped
- 1 teaspoon parsley , finely chopped

To make:

Combine the dressing ingredients and set aside. Allow to come to room temperature.

Quarter tomatoes.

Slice cucumbers carefully.

Break up the greens and alternate layers in two salad bowls.

Lay several tomato and cucumber slices arranged on top of the greens.

Shake the dressing gently to mix all ingredients and drizzle over the top of the greens and tomatoes.

Sprinkle liberally with sunflower seed.

Note. Tomatoes are very healthy; chock full of a nutrient called lycopene. The lycopene is a very good "anti-cancer" booster, but it requires either being cooked or a small amount of oil to be absorbed well. The olive oil in this salad dressing is actually a booster that will help the tomatoes to offer even more health benefits.

Creamy Broccoli and Cauliflower Salad

The tastes of raw broccoli and cauliflower were just made for summer time. This is an amazing taste treat and is also remarkably healthy. Cruciferous vegetables such as broccoli and cauliflower are not only heart healthy but may actually combat cancer and are high in vitamin A.

As quickly as this salad can be created and tasty as it is you may well find the perfect way to assure that your children will eat their veggies even in the summer time. The creamy taste of the salad comes from the slight amount of sour cream, but if you're concerned with calories, you'll get the same taste from a low fat sour cream. In order to create this salad, a small amount of milk can be used to thin the dressing slightly if needed.

You will need:

- One head of broccoli- chopped (not the stems)
- One head of cauliflower, cored and chopped
- 1/2 pound of precooked bacon,(about six slices) fried and chopped or crumbled
- 1/8 cup green onion very finely chopped
- 1/2 cup frozen green peas, thawed, but not cooked

- 1/2 cup grated cheddar cheese
- 1 cup mayonnaise or salad dressing
- 1/2 cup sour cream

To make:

Combine sour cream and Salad Dressing and thin slightly with milk till consistency of a thick salad dressing.

Combine all remaining ingredients and toss together in bowl.

Pour salad dressing over and toss lightly.

Allow to sit in refrigerator so that your flavors can begin to blend slightly before you serve the salad.

Hearty Summer Salad

Brunch or summertime meals can be difficult for those who are gluten intolerant or eat a gluten free diet. Cookouts often   mean that you're getting foods such as hamburgers which incorporate gluten laden ingredients and may also require buns. Gluten free can be a bit more difficult when trying to whip up a cool and easy summertime meal which doesn't require a lot of cooking.

This chickpea and black eyed pea salad is amazingly healthy and refreshing for those days when you just can't even look at the stove. High in protein and in fiber, you'll be well nourished while getting a break from the day to day cooking grind on those hot summer days.

You will need:

- 2 of the 15 oz. cans chickpeas
- 2 of the15 oz. cans black-eyed peas
- 2-15 oz. cans artichoke hearts
- 4 large tomatoes
- ½ large onion
- 3 large fresh garlic cloves
- ¼ cup olive oil
- ½ cup balsamic vinegar

- A few pinches parsley
- Fresh ground salt
- Pepper to taste
- 1/4 cup green olives
- 1/4 teaspoon dried basil

To make:

Drain the beans and add to a bowl.

Chop the artichoke hearts into 8 pieces each and add to the mixture.

Chop tomatoes or dice them into pieces.

Dice your onion and add to the mixture.

Crush the garlic and mince it very finely.

Drain olives and add to the mixture.

Chop the parsley finely.

Add the basil.

Mix your vinegar and olive oil To make a lovely topping.

Drizzle the dressing over the top.

Allow to cool in the refrigerator to blend your flavors for about an hour.

Appetizers and Snacks

It's difficult at times to find gluten free snacks and treats that you can serve at the afternoon Super Bowl Party or just for a quick snack. Most of the processed foods have come into contact with gluten in some way. If you're concerned about making sure that you're not going to be touched by a gluten product or you'd simply like to know how To make your own gluten free treats for a party, we've got a special section of snacks and appetizers for you to create.

Chicken wings are one of our favorite treats. If you're like us, the taste is great and a few of those delectable little bites are just right for an afternoon snack or a small finger food to be served up while you watch the big game. Two different varieties of chicken wings, each of them gluten free are offered here.

Our Chicken Wing recipes have it all. Great taste, lower fat, and just the right amount of heat.

Garlic and Parmesan Chicken Wings

You will need:

- One small can parmesan cheese (8 ounces)
- 1 teaspoon garlic powder
- 2 teaspoons sea salt, ground finely
- 1 stick margarine
- 1/2 teaspoon pepper
- 2 tablespoons corn meal
- 4 pounds chicken wings, cut up into pieces, with tips discarded

To make:

Preheat oven to 400 degrees

Place all ingredients except the margarine and chicken wings into a plastic zip lock bag

Shake to blend ingredients.

Lightly roll chicken wing into margarine and dip into the seasoning.

Place on foil lined cookie or baking sheet.

Sprinkle remaining seasonings over the top of your chicken wings and drizzle with margarine.

Bake at 400 until browned and completely done, approximately 30 minutes in preheated oven.

Test with meat thermometer to ensure proper temperature.

Hot and Spicy Chicken Wings

A little on the spicy side, you'll want to ensure that you have some milk or tomato juice on hand for those who may be affected by the heat in these.

You will need:

- 2 ounces of Louisiana hot sauce or hot pepper sauce
- 1/4 cup of ketchup
- 1/4 cup brown sugar
- 1 stick butter
- 1 teaspoon garlic powder
- sea salt grinder
- freshly ground pepper

To make:

Layer chicken wings on foil covered baking sheet. Brush lightly with butter and season to taste with salt and pepper.

Mix the remaining ingredients together and thoroughly brush over chicken wings.

Bake at 400 approximately 30-40 minutes until done

through.

Tips on "Snackable" Treats

Did you know that the FDA of the United States considers that fruits which have been frozen are comparable in nutrition to those which are fresh and they allow frozen fruit to be labeled as fresh fruit and considered to be healthy. Frozen fruit is already washed and is ready to eat.

Fruit is naturally gluten free and the cleaning the prepping has already been done for you. To enjoy a fast To make treat, take several of your favorites and add them to a smoothie. The phytonutrients as well as the fiber are incredibly good for you, in some cases even helping to detox the body and to give you some amazing nutrients and health benefits. Many fruits actually help to fight cancers of various types and can be used to protect your long term health.

Fruit is gluten free in most cases and it's just plain good for you. Snack on some fresh fruit or even frozen in order to stave off hunger and get a fast and easy gluten free snack.

Gluten Free Conserves and Relishes

Sometimes it's difficult to buy things like cranberry sauce and various types of relish which are not gluten free or aren't guaranteed not to have come into contact with gluten on machinery. Making your own eliminates that risk and gives you a fresher and more delicious product. One of the hardest things to find is a relish that doesn't have additives or glutens such as you will find in many of the different processed relishes and conserves. It's easy to create your own from fresh fruits and vegetables as well as to add other ingredients which are healthy and natural. Why take a chance on the jarred or canned items when you can make your own very easily and in a relatively short amount of time.

Raw Salsa

Salsa is one of our favorite things. Having had some contact with other ethnic groups over time, we've found that most Hispanics do not use the kind of salsa that we do, but rather make it fresh and raw at nearly every meal. We became very accustomed to this kind of salsa and really prefer it to the jarred variety. This recipe for raw salsa is heart healthy, free of gluten and absolutely delicious.

Home Made Spicy Salsa

You will need:

- 6 Roma or other meaty tomatoes
- 6 green onions
- 2 cloves of garlic
- 1 jalapeno
- 1 can chopped green chilies
- Handful of chopped cilantro
- 1 chopped bell pepper
- 1 teaspoon fresh lime juice
- 1/4 teaspoon ground sea salt
- Dash of pepper

To make:

Chop the tomatoes into small squares.

Finely chop remaining ingredients except for the jalapeno and add to the mixture.

Determine how hot you would like your salsa to be. Add one quarter, one half or one full jalapeno, depending upon your preference for heat.

Remove the seeds and chop the pepper finely, adding the portion that you would like.

Refrigerate your salsa for about 2 hours to allow the flavors to blend nicely.

Cranberry Conserve

Cranberry conserve is an old style way to use cranberries. It's a great changeover from the old jellied cranberry sauce that many people serve at the holiday. In our house, there is no such thing as a cranberry sauce that comes from a can. The risk that some of these items have come in contact with gluten is one that we would prefer not to take.

While this is wonderful at the holidays, it's also a super addition to nearly any meal and tastes great when used on burgers for a fresh new style. This is an old Amish recipe which has been rewritten To make it a bit easier To make and to store.

You will need:

- 4 cups of fresh cranberries
- 2 large oranges-sliced
- 1 cup chopped raisins (* you may prefer the golden variety
- of raisins)
- 2 cups of water
- 3 cups pure cane sugar
- 1/2 cup chopped nuts (optional, and we normally omit

- these. If you know of anyone with a nut allergy, avoid them).

To make:

Slice the oranges and discard the seeds

Grind the fresh cranberries and oranges, in a blender or chopper

Transfer it to a heavy sauce pan and add the water.

Cook the fruit rather quickly on a higher fire, being careful to prevent scorching.

Add sugar and raisins. Cook the mix over medium to low heat, stirring the conserve very often, until it begins to thicken.

This freezes very well and can be kept in the refrigerator for up to 14 days.

Gluten Free Desserts - Yes, They Can be Healthy

Healthy gluten free desserts are recipes are much sought after. In many cases, getting chocolate means that it is accompanied by other things that those who need to stay strictly gluten free cannot eat. We can't stress enough that you are going to need to really review cans and ingredients to ensure that your cocoa and other items have not been made on shared equipment and in places where wheat or gluten is present in tiny amounts.

In many cases, although we're uncertain why it is so, the brand names will be made on shared equipment while those which are not major brands will be cleaner and less likely to have contaminants. Check every label carefully to ensure that your products are gluten free and have not had the chance of being contaminated by other products which may contain gluten.

Hot Chocolate Pudding

Not only delicious, but also quite healthy with its touch of cocoa powder, containing phytonutrients that are actually proven to combat some types of cancer, your dessert will be luscious and nutritional, while at the same time being gluten free.

Hot Chocolate pudding is one of the most delicious desserts that you're going to find. It's easy To make and takes about 15 minutes from start to finish.

You will need:

- 2/3 cup pure cane sugar
- 2 tablespoons of corn starch
- pinch of salt
- 1 and 1/2 cups canned milk
- 1 and 1/2 cups water
- 4 egg yolks, slightly beaten
- 1/2 tsp. real vanilla
- 6 ounce bar of Hershey's Dark chocolate
- 1 tsp. Hershey's cocoa

To make:

Combine your sugar, the corn starch and the salt.

Adding about a fourth of a cup of milk, make a very smooth paste-like substance.

Add the remainder of the milk and your egg yolks, stirring til completely blended.

Put the pan over medium heat stirring constantly until it begins to thicken.

Pour into dessert cups and allow to set up about ten minutes.

Transfer into refrigerator or serve warm with a bit of cocoa sifted lightly over the top.

FAST and Easy Gluten Free Rice Pudding

Rice pudding, particularly warm rice pudding is a favorite of nearly everyone who tastes it. Topped with cinnamon it becomes a very healthy ending to your gluten free meal.

You will need:

- 4 egg yolks
- 2/3 cup granulated sugar
- 3 cups of milk
- 2 tablespoons of corn starch
- 1/2 tsp. pure vanilla extract
- 1/4 cup raisins (optional)
- 3/4 cups of instant rice
- dash of cinnamon

To make the rice pudding:

Make the instant rice in the microwave according to package directions. When making it during the last minute of cooking drop in the raisins into the rice to steam and soften them.

In a saucepan, combine the cornstarch, the sugar, and the egg yolks.

Stir until smooth, adding a slight amount of milk as necessary to thin the mixture down to a smooth paste.

Add the remaining milk and stir to combine all ingredients.

Cook over low heat for approximately 12 minutes until the mixture thickens. Do not boil.

Remove from heat and allow cooling approximately 5 minutes.

Drain any remaining water from the rice and raisins.

Combine the rice with the pudding mixture and spoon into dessert dishes.

Dust the top with cinnamon if desired.

Chocolate Fondue Dessert

Dark chocolate has made some big news recently for the fact that it is one of the newest--and the most taste tempting heart healthy foods. Dark chocolate keeps more of the flavonoids than the other varieties. New research is telling us that dark chocolate with its flavonoid content can help to keep your heart healthy and to prevent some types of cardiovascular diseases. Fortunately dark chocolate, which is rich in flavonoids is not rich in gluten--and remains one of the most delicious foods that you can eat which is gluten free.

Obviously that doesn't mean that you can ignore the high calorie content and dash to the store to get yourself a ton of dark chocolate to the exclusion of other kinds of food, but it does mean that when eaten in moderation as part of a healthy diet, dark chocolate can help you to stay healthier in the long term.

Dark Chocolate Fondue

You will need:

- 12 ounces Dark Chocolate finely chopped
- 3/4 cup heavy Whipping Cream

- Fresh strawberries
- Fresh pineapple
- Fresh blueberries
- Sliced bananas
- Fresh sliced apples

To make:

Heat the whipping cream until very warm and drop the chocolate into the whipping cream.

Allow all chocolate to melt thoroughly and stir til smooth, but do not allow boiling.

Keep warm over a pot of warm water in a double boiler and using toothpicks or bamboo skewers and dip the fresh fruit into the chocolate pot.

Gluten Free Chocolate Cake

Also called by some, gluten free soufflé, this is one of the most decadent desserts that you will create which is gluten free. One taste and you're absolutely in love. Much more like a chocolate soufflé than it is a cake; the taste is out of this world. The cocoa adds some antioxidants to your dessert, keeping you healthier and helping to stave off some long term disease processes.

You will need:

- 2 sticks of butter (you must use real butter for this recipe, not margarine which is slightly more watery)
- 1/4 cup Hershey's unsweetened cocoa, plus one teaspoon for dusting the pan
- 8 ounces of bitter, mildly sweetened chocolate, chopped into fine pieces
- 5 eggs
- 1 and 1/4 cups heavy whipping cream
- 1 cup pure cane sugar
- 1/2 cup sour cream
- 1/4 cup powdered sugar

To create the cake:

Preheat your oven to 350 degrees Fahrenheit

Butter a spring form pan measuring 9 inches.

Melt the butter and combine with the quarter cup of heavy cream until it is all melted.

Add the chocolate bars and allow melting. Stir to smooth the mixture and remove it from the heat.

Beat eggs, sugar and cocoa into the chocolate into the buttered pan, add the batter you've just created and bake until the entire mixture is set and puffed up. It will take about 40 minutes to cook completely.

Allow to cool approximately 40 minutes to an hour before you try to unmold the cake.

Beat the sour cream and the confectioners' sugar with the remaining heavy cream and serve as a sauce.

Decadent does not even begin to describe this dessert, which is lovely enough to serve to guests at a holiday dinner.

Baked Apples

With walnuts which are heart healthy, as well as the cinnamon, these can be a healthy part of your diet. Walnuts which contain the omega fatty acids are a good part of a healthy diet. Desserts don't have to be unhealthy. While the butter adds a small amount of saturated fat to your diet, it is so slight as to be negligible.

You will need:

- 4 apples, preferably Cortland or Spies
- 1/4 cup brown sugar
- 5 teaspoons water
- 1/4 teaspoon cinnamon
- 2 tbsp. real butter, cut into slices
- Walnuts or pecans for garnish, as desired

To make baked apples:

Preheat the oven to 375 degrees.

Core the apples, removing the seeds and slice the bottom off so that they lay flat in the baking dish.

Place each apple in the pan.

Drop a small pat of butter inside each apple.

Mix the brown sugar and the water To make a slightly thick syrup.

Drip the syrup over the apples and bake them for approximately 20-30 minutes.

Take the sauce from the dish and spoon over the warm apple.

Serve with ice cream or whipped cream if desired.

Coffee Chocolate Mousse

Chocolate mousse is another of those decadent dessert treats that will leave you feeling very satisfied. You're not going to know that you're missing gluten at all with desserts like these, which make wonderful desserts for dinner parties or for the perfect holiday meal.

You will need:

- One Hershey's Special (tm) dark bar 8 ounce size
- 3 egg yolks, slightly beaten
- 2 teaspoons instant coffee
- 6 tablespoons sugar
- 2 cups whipping cream

To create the mousse:

Melt your chocolate into a bowl over water or in a double boiler. Stir once in a while until smooth.

In a small pan, whip your egg yolks, coffee powder and 3/4 cup of the whipping cream, as well as 4 tbsp. of granulated sugar.

Heat thoroughly, stirring all the while for about three minutes, but do not allow the mixture to completely boil.

Add the mixture to the chocolate mixture, stirring until smooth and glossy.

Cool completely, refrigerating if necessary for about half an hour.

Using your mixer beat the cream and the remaining sugar until it is forming stiff peaks.

Fold in one third of the chocolate mix, then the second, and finally the third portion of it.

Pour into glass serving bowls and refrigerate until hard.

If desired, garnish with shaved chocolate or sifted cocoa powder.

Gluten Free Tips for Fun Kid Foods

It's difficult to have a child who requires a gluten free diet. In many cases, like their friends, they want to eat "normal" foods which can cause them some long term health problems. If you're one of the millions of moms who have a child requiring a gluten free diet, you can't change what they need, but you can change it To make their diet a bit more fun and interesting.

These ideas are based on some fun facts and some fun ideas for moms which can make meal time just a bit less of a struggle.

Gluten Free Breakfast Idea

Remember the old Dr. Seuss Books. One that was always a favorite was "Green Eggs and Ham." Make a child's sleepover a lot more fun and cover the fact that your child isn't eating the typical cereal by making a healthy and a fun breakfast of Green Eggs and Ham.

Just a few drops of food coloring will create a very

festive meal of green eggs and ham, keeping your child--
and his or her prospective company--away from the fact
that there are not the typical sugary cereals at the
breakfast table. Additionally you're adding some real
nutritional value and keeping them clear of high sugar
breakfast foods.

To turn scrambled eggs green, you'll want to use blue
food coloring, while the green works well on the ham
(turkey ham is better). Just a drop will do the job.

Gluten Free Chocolate Chip Cookies

Kids love chocolate chip cookies, but finding one that is gluten free and allows your child to enjoy the treats that other kids take for granted isn't always an easy task. Even some chocolate chips are processed on equipment that is not always free of the allergen that troubles them.

One answer to this is using buckwheat flour to create recipes. Despite its name, buckwheat is not true wheat. It is gluten free, according to the Celiac disease website and offers a lot of protein and iron on top of being gluten free.

Creating chocolate chip cookies from buckwheat, which is a good substitute for traditional flour makes them a tiny bit heavier but allows your kids to have the treat that they want, and you want to give them.

You will need:

- 1 and 1/4 cup buckwheat flour
- 1/2 tsp. soda
- 1/2 tsp. salt
- 1 stick of butter

- 1/4 cup dark brown sugar
- 1/2 tsp. vanilla extract
- 1 egg
- 1 cup chocolate chips (remember to check the package to ensure they are gluten free)

To make:

Combine the dry ingredients except the sugar

Whip together softened butter, egg and sugar

Mix the sugar mixture with the remaining dry ingredients and mix thoroughly.

Stir in chocolate chips

Drop by rounded teaspoons onto a lined cookie sheet.

Bake at 375 degrees for 9-12 minutes.

Crock Pot Cookery and Gluten Free?

One of the questions that is most frequently asked is can I make gluten free recipes in the crock pot. The answer to that is a resounding yes. Most soups and stews are naturally gluten free, using only meats and vegetables. Your favorite recipes of any kind can be made in the crock pot to give you some easy ways to create a meal ahead of time.

Adapting recipes for your slow cooker.

Whether you are cooking traditional foods or gluten free foods, there are times when you want to prepare your food ahead of time and have it ready to go when you arrive at home. In most cases, vegetable and meat stews are going to be easier to prepare and can be made ahead of time to be ready for a hot meal if you're using a crock pot. Soups and stews can have all of the preparation work accomplished the night before and be placed in the crock pot to cook away while you do other things.

Most recipes can be adapted for the crock pot, offering a great way to leave your hands free in meal preparation. The advantages of the crock pot are that they offer you better meals, which are going to be healthier in nature and lower in fats than most of the fast food choices you might make.

Here are a few tips for changing your recipes to crock pot ready recipes.

Bear in mind that if you're going to be using frozen veggies, they only need about half hour, so add them to your recipes for the last 40 minutes of cooking.

Soak dried items such as beans or lentils for an hour or so prior to adding them to the crock pot.

If the recipes require pasta, even gluten free pasta, that too should only be added in the last hour of cooking time.

Bear in mind that you want to lower the liquid amounts in crock pot cooking. You will want to lower them by about one quarter of the overall liquid recipe since the lid doesn't allow for a vast amount of evaporation.

When using the crock pot, layering the veggies on the

bottom and adding the meat to the top is the best plan of action.

If your recipe takes about 30 minutes cook time, it will take about 3 hours on high, 4 hours on medium, and 6 hours on low in the crock pot.

Restaurant Foods on a Gluten Free Diet

Eating out always has the potential to be difficult, but it can be particularly so when you are on any type of a restricted diet. Typically any meal that offers gravy is going to use a roux to thicken it, so make sure that you ask before you order that Sunday roast at a restaurant.

Many places today cater to gluten free people and do have a special menu that they can offer which allows for gravy and sauces which are made from corn flour rather than roux as a thickening agent.

Prior to heading out to a new restaurant a phone call may be in order to find out what kind of foods are available on the menu rather than hoping you find something you may be able to eat and finding out that you're wrong.

Nearly every restaurant serves fresh fruit of some type, but you'll want to be sure there is something else there that you can make a meal of rather than leaving it to chance.

If you find yourself in a restaurant on the spur of the moment, there are some foods that usually do not require the addition of anything which may be gluten laden.

Some choices that you can make which are typically gluten free in the restaurants (although do ask to be sure) include:

- Roast turkey
- Broiled Chicken
- Pork Chops
- Broiled Steaks
- Fresh steamed veggies

Desserts are going to be the most difficult to get when you are on a gluten free diet, but bear in mind that your selections can include fruit salads, as well as crème brulee, along with nearly any type of pudding which is typically made with corn flour as opposed to a flour thickening agent.

Make sure that you ask your server and if you do not get a satisfactory answer, do ask to speak with the chef in order to find out what kind of gluten free menu items the restaurant offers.

Tips on Living Gluten Free:

1. Many foods are naturally gluten free. You do not have to shop the fringe to find all gluten free foods. Things like rice noodles, buckwheat, fruits and veggies are gluten free naturally. Use those products and save some money on the cost of buying gluten free.

2. Use common sense. Many companies make a big production and a big payday by touting their foods as gluten free. There is even a gluten free rice. The rice grain is naturally gluten free so make sure you are aware of what foods are gluten free before paying more for a product that may be naturally gluten free.

3. Many stores carry a list of foods that are gluten free. Bigger shopping sites such as Trader Joe's, Wegmans and many other supermarkets will be glad to give you a list of gluten free goods and enable you To make great choices without searching the entire store.

4. Make sure you look for "gluten free" on the label. Gluten free and wheat free are two entirely different things and not all products which are free of wheat are also free of gluten.

5. Buy a few good books. Richard Coppedge, Jr, who is a professor of baking and pastry arts at The Culinary Institute of America is also the author of a book on gluten free baking that may become your new Bible. " Gluten-Free Baking With The Culinary Institute of America: 150 Flavorful Recipes From the World's Premier Culinary College.

6. Some types of oil may have been made on equipment which was shared with gluten containing products. Check the labels of everything, even those foods which you believe should be gluten free. It doesn't hurt to be a little extra careful.

7. Many companies today make foods which are already done and are gluten free. Check them for use in those moments when you need something fast and easy. Gluten free premade meals are available in most regular supermarkets today.

8. Online websites are one of the best places to find gluten free tips and new gluten free recipes. In fact, at last count there were about 5000 gluten free recipe sites which can be used to help you to supplement your meals and to get great substitutions for foods or products that contain gluten.

9. If you live in a small area, supermarkets and even companies such as Amazon are offering online gluten free products that you can order. Typically the shipping prices are quite low and you'll have the products within just a few days. If you live in an area where the supermarket is not large and gluten free products aren't part of what they carry, shopping online can be a life-saver.

10. Rice flour is amazing for fried foods. While it is gritty and often causes problems in bread, the rice flour for use when frying items or making tempura is a wonderful addition because that bit of extra texture is very welcome. Don't rule out rice flour all together when you're cooking because of the grit.

References and Credits

We've made several statements during the course of the book which promote the use of broccoli, cauliflower, and other cruciferous vegetables being used in gluten free cooking to aid in detoxifying the body and to assist in adding fiber to the diet. These statements are made using references from the Pub Med materials and the Nutritional Journal references which can be found below.

Ambrosone CB, Tang L. Cruciferous vegetable intake and cancer prevention: role of nutrigenetics. Cancer Prev Res (Phila Pa). 2009 Apr;2(4):298-300.

Angeloni C, Leoncini E, Malaguti M, et al. Modulation of phase II enzymes by sulforaphane: implications for its cardioprotective potential. J Agric Food Chem. 2009 Jun 24;57(12):5615-22.

Banerjee S, Wang Z, Kong D, et al. 3,3'-Diindolylmethane enhances chemosensitivity of multiple chemotherapeutic agents in pancreatic cancer. 3,3'-Diindolylmethane enhances chemosensitivity of multiple chemotherapeutic agents in pancreatic cancer.

Bhattacharya A, Tang L, Li Y, et al. Inhibition of bladder cancer development by allyl isothiocyanate. Carcinogenesis. 2010 Feb;31(2):281-6.

Bryant CS, Kumar S, Chamala S, et al. Sulforaphane induces cell cycle arrest by protecting RB-E2F-1 complex in epithelial ovarian cancer cells. Molecular Cancer 2010, 9:47.

Christopher B, Sanjeez K, Sreedhar C, et al. Sulforaphane induces cell cycle arrest by protecting RB-E2F-1 complex in epithelial ovarian cancer cells. Molecular Cancer Year: 2010 Vol: 9 Issue: 1 Pages/record No.: 47.

Clarke JD, Dashwood RH, Ho E. Multi-targeted prevention of cancer by sulforaphane. Cancer Lett. 2008 Oct 8;269(2):291-304.

Cornelis MC, El-Sohemy A, Campos H. GSTT1 genotype modifies the association between cruciferous vegetable intake and the risk of myocardial infarction. Am J Clin Nutr. 2007 Sep;86(3):752-8.

Hu J, Straub J, Xiao D, et al. Phenethyl isothiocyanate, a cancer chemopreventive constituent of cruciferous vegetables, inhibits cap-dependent translation by regulating the level and phosphorylation of 4E-BP1. Cancer Res. 2007 Apr 15;67(8):3569-73.

Jiang H, Shang X, Wu H, et al. Combination treatment with resveratrol and sulforaphane induces apoptosis in human U251 glioma cells. Neurochem Res. 2010 Jan;35(1):152-61.

Special Thanks to WHFoods for their valuable information on broccoli, cauliflower and other cruciferous vegetables as well as the reference materials to point us in the right direction.

The American Journal of Clinical Nutrition was an invaluable resource in the creation of this book. Find them online at http://ajcn.nutrition.org/

Lightning Source UK Ltd.
Milton Keynes UK
UKOW05f2338101216
289652UK00030B/1221/P